The International Librar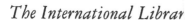

COMMON SENSE AND ITS CULTIVATION

Founded by C. K. Ogden

The International Library of Psychology

COGNITIVE PSYCHOLOGY
In 21 Volumes

I	The Psycho-Analysis of Artistic Vision and Hearing	*Ehrenzweig*
II	A Source Book of Gestalt Psychology	*Ellis*
III	Common Sense and its Cultivation	*Hankin*
IV	The Nature of Learning	*Humphrey*
V	Eidetic Imagery and Typological Methods of Investigation	*Jaensch*
VI	The World of Colour	*Katz*
VII	Principles of Gestalt Psychology	*Koffka*
VIII	Colour and Colour Theories	*Ladd-Franklin*
IX	Sense-Perception and Matter	*Lean*
X	Invention and the Unconscious	*Montmasson*
XI	Psychology and Education	*Ogden*
XII	Human Speech	*Paget*
XIII	The Gestalt Theory and the Problem of Configuration	*Petermann*
XIV	Surprise and the Psycho-Analyst	*Reik*
XV	The Psychology of a Musical Prodigy	*Révész*
XVI	Biological Memory	*Rignano*
XVII	The Psychology of Reasoning	*Rignano*
XVIII	The Effects of Music	*Schoen*
XIX	Analysis of Perception	*Smythies*
XX	Speech Disorders	*Stinchfield*
XXI	The Psycho-Biology of Language	*Zipf*

COMMON SENSE AND ITS CULTIVATION

HANBURY HANKIN

Foreword by C S Myers

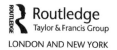

Routledge
Taylor & Francis Group

LONDON AND NEW YORK

First published in 1926 by
Routledge, Trench, Trubner & Co., Ltd.

Reprinted in 1999, 2001 by
Routledge

2 Park Square, Milton Park, Abingdon, Oxon, OX14 4RN

Simultaneously published in the USA and Canada by Routledge

711 Third Avenue, New York, NY 10017

Transferred to Digital Printing 2007

Routledge is an imprint of the Taylor & Francis Group

First issued in paperback 2013

The publishers have made every effort to contact authors/copyright holders
of the works reprinted in the *International Library of Psychology*.
This has not been possible in every case, however, and we would
welcome correspondence from those individuals/companies
we have been unable to trace.

These reprints are taken from original copies of each book. In many cases
the condition of these originals is not perfect. The publisher has gone to
great lengths to ensure the quality of these reprints, but wishes to point
out that certain characteristics of the original copies will, of necessity, be
apparent in reprints thereof.

British Library Cataloguing in Publication Data
A CIP catalogue record for this book
is available from the British Library

Common Sense and its Cultivation

ISBN 978-0-415-20958-8 (hbk)
ISBN 978-0-415-86436-7 (pbk)

CONTENTS

Chapter.	Page
I—What is Meant by Common Sense ?	1
II—Subconscious Judgment	21
III—Examples of Subconscious Judgment	32
IV—On Abnormal Calculating Power	53
V—Calculating Ability and Intuition	74
VI—Musical Genius	92
VII—Formal Reasoning and Subconscious Judgment	102
VIII—Experts as Directors of Commercial Companies	133
IX—Experts as Business Men	145
X—Confidence Tricks and their Explanation	152
XI—The Mental Limitations of the Globe-Trotter	164
XII—Opposition to New Ideas	172
XIII—The Critical Faculty of the Practical Man	194
XIV—On Educational Systems	204
XV—The Mental Ability of the Quakers	238
XVI—The Teaching of Morality	268
Index	285

FOREWORD

Hitherto I have invariably declined an author's invitation to write an introduction to his book. The task has always appeared to me as singularly uncongenial, and as one in which, judging from the introductions which I have come across, I should be little likely to succeed. Moreover, I regard it as an objectionable survival of the bygone days of patronage ; the merits of a book should be left to speak for themselves.

But in the present instance, there were exceptional circumstances to be taken into consideration. The author is dealing with a subject which is not his own. Anyone now thinks himself entitled, without previous training in the subject, to write on psychology ; wherefore its extreme interest and its extreme difficulty threaten to bring it into ridicule as a science. On the other hand it has reaped undoubted benefits from certain "outsiders" who, approaching it from a fresh standpoint untrammelled by tradition, have "seen most of the game." Despite a certain exaggeration and want of balance, and a laxity of terminology and scientific procedure, such men of genius as Freud and Jung, have unquestionably given an enormous impetus to the progress of psychology.

Similarly, Dr Hankin's attractive book appears to me well worthy both of expert and of popular consideration. His aim is to distinguish and to oppose the two broad lines of intellectual advance. We may arrive at an idea or discovery by inspiration, or at a judgment or decision by intuition ; in either case we have no knowledge as to how the result is suddenly attained. On the other hand we may attain it slowly by careful reasoning, when we are able to trace the various steps involved. Along the one line success is attributable to unconscious genius or to common sense ; along the other line to a series of conscious processes directed by instinctive talent or else by sheer intellectual effort. As a nation, we have believed rather in genius and common sense ; these have chiefly characterised our progress in science and business.

For the purpose of exposition Dr Hankin may appear to have exaggerated the isolation and opposition between these two instruments of the creative imagination. But his object has been to stress their undoubted differences and to support his novel thesis that genius and intuition are likely to be hampered by allowing education in pre-adolescent years to be governed too exclusively by native interests, to the neglect of hard conscious efforts directed to the mastery of relatively uninteresting material, much of which will soon pass into oblivion, thus ceasing to clog conscious activity in later life by the accumulation of the products of that activity.

I have probably said enough to arouse the interest of the expert and of the general public in this fascinating book. Although, as Dr Hankin admits, the book cannot always claim psychological precision, it well merits general attention ; for it will make the reader think.

CHARLES S. MYERS.

PREFACE

There is a widespread desire to know more of the nature of common sense, in what it consists, to what degree it is present in persons of different mental habits, what conditions are favourable or otherwise to its development and, lastly, whether its development may be stimulated by any practical changes in our educational methods. It is hoped that the facts recorded in this book will throw light on such questions.

Signs are not wanting of discontent with our present system of education. In current literature we find a psychologist writing of the ordinary mind-wrecking processes that take place in schools, a doctor of the evils of over-education, a man of science asserting that our universities are destructive of originality, and a philosopher that our educational methods, whatever their matter, are fundamentally vicious in their manner. Above all this there is a suspicion that education does little or nothing towards the development of common sense. Hence it need cause no surprise if our study leads to serious criticisms of the ordinary present day school curriculum.

My thanks are due to the editor for permission to reprint an article that appeared in *Science Progress* for April, 1922, dealing with the mental ability of the Quakers, and also to Messrs Butterworth and Co. for their permission to incorporate extracts from my book,

Mental Limitations, which was published in India in 1920.

Dr Myers has put me under a great obligation by contributing a foreword. It seems only fair to say that since he read the manuscript, several additions have been made to it, some of which it did not seem worth while to submit to him.

E. HANBURY HANKIN.

January, 1925.

CHAPTER I

WHAT IS MEANT BY COMMON SENSE ?

An example of common sense—Instances of want of common sense—Subconscious judgment—The business instinct—Histories of business men.

" Common sense " is a term used with so many different meanings that it will be well before attempting to define it to consider a large number of examples of mental effort in which it was present and also other examples in which it was lacking. We may begin with the following trivial incident related in connection with the late Sir Gabriel Stokes. He was a man of science distinguished alike for his mathematical ability, his discoveries in physics and a singular deficiency in ordinary conversational powers. At a party held in his house in Cambridge it once happened that a guest remarked to Lady Stokes that two men were present who had not spoken a single word the whole evening. " One of them must be my husband. Come along and let us see who is the other," replied Lady Stokes, thus giving, at a moment's notice, a suitable and sensible reply to an unexpected remark. This may be described as a common-sense reply. How did she do it ? It is no explanation though no doubt a fact, to say that she had had much social experience. What we have to investigate is how such experience enabled her to at once hit on a satisfactory reply without taking time to consciously weigh *pros* and *cons* or to make a choice between different possible answers, and why " on the spur of the moment " the right reply came instantly to her lips.   The main purpose of this book is to investigate the mental processes by which, as in the incident just related, we arrive at sensible decisions without having the least conscious knowledge of how we do so.   In the practical affairs of life such powers are perhaps the most useful as they are the most remarkable and the least studied of our mental faculties.

One may look in vain in current books on psychology for explanations or descriptions of common sense, though full accounts are given of the obsessions, delusions or complexes by which our common sense or our conscious reasoning may alike be vitiated.   Even the conception of common sense appears to be outside the purview of those extreme followers of Freud who, mistaking the misfortunes of the subconscious mind for its functions, think that nothing is worth noticing unless it can be brought into relation with affairs of sex.   On my putting a question on an allied subject to such a psychologist, he replied to me that all mental work of the subconscious mind is " non-rational."   Such an opinion was very unexpected as this gentleman had just published a book in which he quoted with approval a statement that the subconscious mind is capable of everything that we understand by the term " reason."   His reply led me to submit to him instances of those arithmetical prodigies who can solve difficult problems instantly without their having the least idea as to how they arrive at their results. Such instances seemed to furnish a convincing proof that the subconscious mind is capable of intellectual work. But in his letter in reply he asserted that such calculations are " automatic " and that the results are arrived at by " intuition." My next enquiry was whether a calculating prodigy doing a cube root for the first time subconsciously, would find an intuition ready made in his head to help him.* He thereupon put an end to our correspondence, informing me that to explain his views he would have to refer to the original German, which, he stated, would be beyond my powers to understand. Why my correspondent should thus modestly conceal his ignorance by using thrionic† phrases about automatic actions and intuitions is a matter of some interest. His book, to which reference has been made, as regards the special subjects in which the researches of Freud are of importance, is admirably and clearly written. But as regards other branches of psychology it is obscure and perhaps misleading. The reason for this appears to be connected with the fact that if an emotion is normally repressed it has to stay repressed if one is to retain one's mental equilibrium. Excessive contemplation of the relations of the sexes is unpleasant to the normally constituted mind. If the implied repression is removed there is a liability for the emotions connected with sex to " take charge," as the sailors say, and lead to a frame of mind in which nothing is thought to be explained or worth explaining unless it can be

---

* This question will be discussed in Chapters IV and V.

† θρῖον, a figleaf.

brought into relation with sex instincts. To such a person, the idea that the subconscious mind can perform intellectual work other than what is involved in recognising a particular kind of symbol in any object whose length is greater than its breadth, may well appear as a sort of desecration.

The incident related in the opening paragraph of this chapter is by no means sufficient to illustrate all that is commonly meant by common sense. We may learn more by considering some examples of mental effort in which common sense was conspicuously lacking.

When the philosopher Herbert Spencer was once present at an opera, his enjoyment was entirely marred by the behaviour of the minor characters. " That serving men and waiting maids," he wrote, " should be made poetical and prompted to speak in *recitative*, because their masters and mistresses happened to be in love, was too conspicuous an absurdity." We may surmise that Herbert Spencer's great reasoning power was given him by some wayward fairy who added to it the curse that he should always use it. This he did, as we shall see, both on occasions when common sense rather than formal reason was called for and also when, as on the present occasion, he would have been better advised merely to look on and enjoy himself. The lack of common sense displayed on this occasion was due to his having reasoned on a too narrow range of data. Had he consulted a writer of plays and operas he might have learnt that prosaic replies in nineteenth century English by waiting maids or serving men would have destroyed the emotional appeal made by the rest of the opera.

In his younger days Herbert Spencer once heard that a friend of his was engaged to be married and thereupon sent him a letter of congratulation which consisted chiefly in a disquisition on marriage in which he expressed such sentiments as the following :—

" There should be a thorough recognition on both sides of the equality of rights, and no amount of power should ever be claimed by one party greater than that claimed by the other. The present relationship as existing between husband and wife, where one claims a command over the actions of the other, is nothing more than *a remnant of the old leaven of slavery*. It is necessarily destructive of refined love ; for *how can a man continue to regard as his type of the ideal a being whom he has, by denying an equality of privilege with himself, degraded to something below himself ?* To me the exercise of command on the part of a husband seems utterly repugnant to genuine love, and I feel sure that a man of generous feeling has too much sympathy with the dignity of his wife to think of dictating to her, and that no woman of truly noble mind will submit to be dictated to."

Spencer, in his autobiography, comments on this letter that " It seems proper to remark that at the age of 73, one must not be held bound to *all* the opinions one expressed at the age of 24." A young lady once wrote to a lady of my acquaintance in almost identical terms about the indignity of obeying one's husband. She had an excuse for her opinions that was lacking to the philosopher in that she was a militant suffragette and so perhaps it was natural that she should conceive of matrimonial bliss as a state of armed neutrality. The lady who received this letter was at the time engaged to be married and on getting married discovered that by making a strict rule of obeying her husband, it became easy to negotiate the exceptions when it was necessary to do the contrary.

Both the philosopher and the suffragette argued on a too narrow range of data.

Tennyson once wrote a poem called " The Vision of Sin," in which occurs the lines :—

" Every moment dies a man,
Every moment one is born."

When this poem was published it came into the hands of the mathematician Babbage, the well-known inventor of a calculating machine of great scientific interest rather than of practical use. He thereupon wrote to the poet as follows :—

" In your otherwise beautiful poem, there is a verse which reads :—

" Every moment dies a man,
Every moment one is born."

" It must be manifest that were this true, the population of the world would be at a standstill. In truth the rate of birth is slightly in excess of that of death.

" I would suggest that in the next edition of your poem, you have it read :—

" Every moment dies a man,
Every moment 1 1/16 is born."

" Strictly speaking this is not correct. The actual figure is a decimal so long that I cannot get it in the line, but I believe 1 1/16 will be sufficiently accurate for poetry. I am, etc."

The mathematician, like the philosopher and the suffragette, argued on a too narrow range of data and hence was wanting in common sense. A further insight into the nature of this mental defect is furnished by the following letter received by the late Sir Charles Hawtrey —and quoted by him in his autobiography as an example of the wild financial schemes that were sometimes submitted to him :—*

" Knowing you have had some interest in the fur business, I take the liberty of presenting you with what seems to me a most wonderful business proposition, and in which no doubt you will take a lively interest, and perhaps wire me the amount of stock that you want to subscribe towards the foundation of this company.

" The object of this company is to operate a large cat ranch in or near Oakland where land can be purchased cheap for this purpose.

" To start with, we will collect say about 100,000 cats. Each cat will average about twelve kittens a year. The skins run from 10 cents each for white ones and 75 cents for the pure black. This will give us twelve million skins a year to sell at an average price of 30 cents each, making our revenue about 10,000 dollars gross.

" A man can skin 50 cats per day for 2 dollars. It will take 100 men to operate the ranch, and therefore the net profit will thus be 9,800 dollars per day.

---

* *The truth at last from Charles Hawtrey* (Thornton Butterworth, 1924).

B

" We will feed the cats on rats and will start the rat ranch next door.   The rats multiply four times as fast as the cats, and if we start with one million rats we will have therefore four rats per day for each cat, which will be plenty.

" Now then, we will feed the rats on the carcases of the cats from which the skins have been taken, giving each rat one fourth of a cat.

" It will thus be seen that the business will be self-supporting and automatic all the way through.   The cats will eat the rats, the rats will eat the cats, and we will get the skins.

" Awaiting your prompt reply, and trusting you will appreciate the opportunity that I give you, and which will get you rich quick.

" I remain, etc."

It is unnecessary to emphasise the fact that the absurdity of this scheme is due to its author having argued on a too narrow range of data.   But what we have to consider is that my readers instantly see that the scheme is absurd because their opinion is influenced by a wide range of data.   But these data do not appear to enter their consciousness to any appreciable degree. The readers' appreciation of the absurdity is instantaneous while their appreciation of the reasons for the absurdity is a comparatively slow process.   While some of their reasons can be called into consciousness, it is probable that other reasons remain in their subconscious minds and yet play a part in influencing their opinion. We have now to consider a large number of proofs of different kinds that data stored in the subconscious minds may take part in intellectual processes, the end results of which alone enter consciousness.

The above examples enable us to appreciate another feature of what we call common sense. Common-sense decisions to deserve the name must appear sensible to sensible people. This is only possible if such decisions are based on a sufficiently wide range of data.

In some subjects, for instance in scientific matters, a narrow range of data are all that is required, but these data have to be handled within the domain of consciousness. As an instance we may quote Edison's discovery of quadruplex telegraphy. His problem was to arrange for four messages to travel over a single wire at the same time. While thinking of what the dots and dashes of one message were doing, he had to bear in mind what was happening to the dots and dashes of three other messages. The difficulty was to keep his knowledge of all these events at the same time in the field of consciousness. He says of it : " The problem was of the most difficult and complicated kind, and I bent all my energies toward its solution. It required a peculiar effort of the mind, such as the imagining of eight different things moving simultaneously on a mental plane, without anything to demonstrate their efficiency." The problem was hard reasoning but it was not common sense. The mental effort required appears to have rendered the recalling of unconnected data less easy than usual. For instance, his biographers record that at the time " when notified he would have to pay $12\frac{1}{2}$ per cent.

extra if his taxes in Newark were not at once paid, he actually forgot his own name when asked for it suddenly at the City Hall, lost his place in the line, and the fatal hour striking, had to pay the surcharge after all! "*

Another example of clever formal reasoning may be quoted. The Mogul Emperor Aurungzebe was once at war with a refractory rajah and was endeavouring to surround the latter's territory with his army. One of Aurungzebe's sons seized this opportunity to go into rebellion. He joined forces with this rajah and together they began to advance to attack the Emperor. Aurungzebe, who was of opinion that a wise king should be suspicious even of his own shadow, was well informed, by means of his spies, of his son's intentions. He had but few troops with him at the time and, if he was to save himself, it was imperatively necessary to delay the day of battle. He first bribed the Prince's attendants to represent to their master that success was so certain that he had better at once make arrangements for his coronation. The Prince fell in with the idea and halted for the purpose. Some days respite were thereby obtained. At length messengers came to Aurungzebe telling him the prince was ready to start. He thereupon sent bribes to the prince's astrologers who discovered that the stars were unpropitious and that it was necessary to wait for several more days for an auspicious moment for the battle. When no more delay could be obtained in this way, Aurungzebe wrote

---

* *Edison, His Life and Inventions*, by F. L. Dyer and T. C. Martin (New York, Harper Brothers, 1910).

a letter to his son which he arranged should fall into the hands of the rajah. The rajah opened it and read that it was arranged that, as soon as the battle began, the prince's troops should treacherously attack the rajah. The latter, thinking this was really the prince's intention, deserted him. Aurungzebe had no difficulty in capturing the prince who was sent to the state prison at Gwalior where he passed the rest of his life.

This is an example of clever reasoning over a wide range of data but it was not common sense because it is probable that Aurungzebe considered *pros* and *cons* and was conscious of reasons for each of his decisions. The incident is quoted because, as will be seen in a later chapter, he held typical commonplace opinions on the necessity of " vocational education " for a prince. It seems likely that his son had enjoyed this presumed advantage without, as we have seen, thereby acquiring any trace of common sense.

In the ordinary affairs of life, on the other hand, our judgment is only likely to be right if it is influenced by an enormously wide range of data which are far too many to be dealt with consciously. The data have to exert their influence while still in the subconscious mind. In attempting to solve the problem of cultivating our common sense, the first step must be to discover the nature of the process by which sense impressions are stored in the subconscious mind in such a way as to be available in influencing our opinions. We then have to consider how to train the mind to use such data without recalling them into consciousness.

It will be convenient to speak of "subconscious judgment" to describe a decision in which data present in the subconscious mind play a predominant part. It will be unavoidable to write as if " conscious reasoning " and an act of subconscious judgment were two perfectly distinct mental processes, although, as in the instance of the absurdity of the cat and rat scheme just described, they shade off into one another by gradations that are difficult to recognise.

By way of comparing these two modes of reasoning, let us consider the mental processes involved in discovering a new aniline dye—the work of an expert—and in putting it on the market—the work of a man of business.

The mental work of an expert carrying out a research of this nature consists almost entirely of observation guided by formal reasoning. That is to say his opinions are based on evidence known to his consciousness. His reasoning power is aided by his memory which is highly trained for its special purpose. Facts that he has apparently forgotten readily come back when needed in a reasoned line of argument. His efficiency as an expert depends to a very great extent on the power of calling to mind the data required for his reasoning processes.

But sooner or later in his work he meets with a difficulty that he is unable to solve by any such simple mental process. He then has to wait for an original idea. Such an idea appears to be a product of the subconscious mind ; for it may come to him at the moment of waking, when he finds the idea present in his mind without any conscious effort on his part. Or original ideas may come to him while thinking. They occur instantaneously, as difficulties arise, and occur so rapidly that there is no time for them to have resulted from a formal reasoning process. But such ideas are never accepted by the expert till they have been tested. Indeed his original ideas are usually nothing more than suggestions for new experiments.

The progress of the young expert is one of trial and error. As a rule he only goes right after testing every way, or at least a large number of ways, of going wrong. But, as he gains experience, he may learn to recognise instinctively which of several courses is the best to choose or which is the best method of testing to employ or which line of research is best worth following up. But any such power of instinct or intuition depending on an activity of the subconscious mind is always subordinate to his formal reasoning. " Genius," said Edison, " is one per cent. inspiration and ninety-nine per cent. perspiration."

Supposing that by the application of such mental processes, the new dye has been discovered, the next question to solve is whether it can be made commercially. In attacking this question formal reason still reigns supreme. By such reasoning an estimate has to be made of the cost of manufacture, of the availability of raw materials and the possibilities of using bye-products that may be formed in the process. A wider view of the matter has to be taken than was necessary for discovering the dye, but still the mental process involved is mainly one of conscious reasoning.

Now, suppose it has been discovered how to make the dye on a large scale at a suitable price, and suppose the matter comes into the hands of a business man. As an example, let us imagine that the problem that presents itself is whether it would pay to dissolve the dye in water, put it in bottles and sell it as ink. In the first place the business man has to make an estimate of the cost of bottling and packing and labelling, problems that can be solved by the use of conscious reasoning. But he very soon comes to problems that can not be solved in this way in the time and with the data available. He has to consider what credit to give, what contracts to enter into, whom to appoint, what buildings to rent and what money to spend on advertisements. He must also consider what other inks are in the market, what will be the effects of competition, whether his rivals will cut their prices and so on. If such processes had to be treated by formal reasoning, his progress would be slow and laborious. Vast amounts of data and highly involved arguments would be required. Anyone who knows business men will admit grounds for doubting whether they are capable of highly involved arguments. Usually the business man shows an instinctive dislike for a reasoned argument. For his special problems, that apparently need more reasoning and more data than those treated of by the expert, he brings into play less reasoning and fewer data. Instead of taking more time to settle complicated questions he takes less time than does the expert in settling far simpler affairs. In short, when faced with business problems, the conscious reasoning of the business man goes into the background and is replaced by a mental activity commonly termed the " business instinct." This term is in no sense an explanation. It is a popular term similar to the terms " journalistic instinct " or the " instinct of the statesman " that we find in current literature. Before attempting to consider further the nature of the business instinct, it will be advisable to describe in some detail the mental capacities of the typical man of business.

An acquaintance with business men quickly reveals the fact that a high degree of intelligence is compatible with a singular absence of general knowledge. A financier once puzzled me very much by saying that he used a great deal of higher mathematics in his business. This I explained to him seemed strange, as business men are in the habit of arriving at conclusions so rapidly that there can be no time for calculating. A merchant, I told him, once said to me that the chief part of his business consisted in arriving at important decisions at ten seconds' notice. " So do I," my friend replied, " but I only take one second." To my question whether this was not due to some activity of the subconscious mind, he replied, " I don't know that word. I call it higher mathematics."

It is easy to say that such rapidity was due to practice. But that is not the whole story. The late Lord Raleigh had much practice in experimenting. He was famed as a skilled experimenter. But yet his experience had not given him the gift of rapid decision in such work. It is recorded that when a difficulty occurred in an experiment he preferred not to attempt to solve it at the time but to sleep on it and do something else in the meanwhile. In other matters also he could not be easily induced to give a hasty decision.

A business man once gave me the following account of his career. His father was creditor of a spinning mill that went bankrupt. He persuaded his father to take over the mill and put him in as manager. He knew nothing whatever at the time about cotton. He had never managed a factory of any kind. But he began on this mill and in a short time made it a success. Afterwards he started a flour mill at a time when he knew nothing about flour and then an ice factory when equally ignorant of ice. He then built several more factories. Eventually he sold his concern for a large sum of money and retired from business. His success was partly due to his faculty for choosing the right men to supervise the different departments. He was always quite innocent of either technical skill or expert knowledge. He had forgotten most of what he had learnt at school. He had taken prizes for mathematics but when he became a business man he could not remember the title of a single proposition of Euclid. He even could not define parallel straight lines. He said that parallel lines were lines that were parallel. He could not even attempt the kind of mental exertion needed to think of a definition. So little capable was he of logical presentment that he was quite unable to explain to me the difference between the deferred shares and the ordinary shares in a particular company. All that he could tell me was that this was something that had been settled before the company was formed. But when asked what he thought of these shares as an investment he at once gave definite opinions. The ordinary shares would, in the next three months, he said, rise from 95 to 300 and the deferred shares from about 120 to 1,000. He could give no satisfactory logical reasons for his belief, but, as the event proved, his business instinct had led him to make a remarkably accurate forecast in each case. After his retirement he had no interest in life except gambling, in which pastime he is reputed to have lost the greater part of his fortune.

An American business man once told me his history. He had had an indifferent school education and at an early age had had to shift for himself. He became a clerk on a railway. He found some additional employment for his spare hours and contrived to save money. After a time he threw up his job and moved to a town somewhere in California. He came there without any invitation or offer of employment. He merely trusted to his natural wit to be able to take advantage of anything that turned up. He installed himself in a boarding house. On the day of his arrival it happened that there were stewed onions for dinner. He asked their price and where they came from. The next day he happened to see a number of boxes of onions outside a shop. " How much are they," he asked. " Ten cents a bushel," said the shopman. " Then," said he, " I'll buy the lot." Afterwards, as he assured me, he discovered that this was the only stock of onions in the place. One wonders whether on this point he was not suffering from an inaccurate memory. " What did you know about onions ? " I asked him. " Nothing," he replied. On my asking what he knew about trade he gave me the same reply. He went on with his story. The price of onions went up. He purchased the next available supply from a neighbouring town whence they had to come by ship. He still kept up the price until he received information that more onions were arriving by another route when he at once disposed of all he had at a good profit. The whole of his life history seemed to have been made up of similar incidents. Lack of knowledge that would have checkmated an expert was of no importance to him. He was always ready to turn to a thing about which he knew practically nothing provided his business instinct told him there was a chance of coining money. He was quite interesting to talk to, though totally ignorant of anything he had not dealt with in the way of business.

Both of these business men lacked both the enterprise, the imagination and the knowledge that would be needed for making practical applications of new discoveries. An example of the results of having expert directors on the boards of a commercial company is given by the history of artificial indigo. Briefly it may be stated that some thirty years ago, several chemical processes were known by means of which it was possible to produce indigo in small quantities. It remained to discover a process that would be useful on a large scale. Two German firms of makers of aniline dyes joined forces to carry on a research on this point. A large number of skilled experts were employed who worked at the problem for years without success. After nearly a million pounds had been spent on the research the partnership was dissolved. An expert belonging to one of the firms, however, continued the research. A process was known to him for making one of the parent substances of indigo in which certain chemicals were heated together to a particular degree. The yield thereby produced had hitherto been only a small fraction of what had been hoped and expected. But on this occasion, on repeating the experiment, his thermometer broke. This time, to his astonishment, he found that nearly a hundred per cent. of the desired product had been formed. The result was found to be due to the presence of the mercury that had escaped from the broken thermometer. The main problem was now solved. Further expensive researches were still needed for discovering methods of making in sufficient purity and at a sufficiently low price certain of the chemicals that were needed in the process. When these had been carried out successfully, the firm was in a position to produce synthetic indigo at a price that would undersell the Indian indigo planter. A large factory was thereupon built for the purpose. They considered that they had it in their power to supply the whole of the world's needs of indigo. They decided however to produce only a fraction, if my memory serves me rightly, it was four-fifths of the total amount. Though their patents were perfectly valid and though the success of their process was assured, they recognised the possibility of some other process being discovered. Hence they left one-fifth of the world's supply unsatisfied under the impression that the holder of any new process would take his profits out of the Indian planter instead of out of them. The very distinguished expert who told me this story considered the plan to be highly ingenious and commendable. But it is not a plan that would appeal to a business man, and its unsoundness was proved by the result. A fresh process was discovered by the rival firm, with resulting competition and fall in prices to the benefit, no doubt, of the consumer. In other respects also, as will be seen later, the success of German aniline dye companies seems to be due to their directors having enterprise, knowledge, imagination and also good things to sell, but not to their being well endowed with business instinct.

An important feature of the mental activity that we call the business instinct is the rapidity with which important decisions are often reached. It takes some time to reason out a proposition of Euclid. But matters far more complicated than anything treated of by Euclid may be decided by a business man on the spur of the moment. We are dealing with a more recondite power of the human mind than conscious reasoning. This power of deciding rapidly in business matters is analogous to the power possessed by many doctors of making a rapid diagnosis without, in some cases, being able to give reasons for their decision. In each case we are dealing with rational decisions in which the activity of the subconscious mind plays a larger part than it does in formal reasoning.

CHAPTER II

SUBCONSCIOUS JUDGMENT

Business Instinct—Subconscious diagnosis by doctors—Power
of rapidly judging character or capacity—Refusing credit
on instinctive feeling—Minute sensory impressions affecting
the subconscious mind only—Use of such impressions—
Illustrations.

'However commonplace it may appear to say that a
business man depends on his business instinct, that he
should do so is a fact well worth attention. The main
apparent effort of his education has been to develop
the power of arriving at rational decisions on evidence
present to his consciousness. But when the boy grows
up and becomes a man of business, he constantly has
to arrive at rational decisions for which the evidence is
not available or only partly available to his conscious
mind. Rational decisions of this nature may be described
as being cases of subconscious judgment. We now
have to consider further examples of subconscious judgment and to see how far they resemble the business
instinct.

The first instance to be described is the power of rapid
diagnosis possessed by many medical men. It frequently happens that doctors distinguished for their
power of rapid and accurate diagnosis are unable to
give reasons for the opinions they form. For instance,
a medical man gave me a detailed account of a doctor,

at a hospital where my informant had been a student, who had a power of this kind that was little short of marvellous. A child arrived one day at the hospital very ill. Several members of the staff examined the child carefully, but were unable to discover what was the matter with it. Afterwards the doctor in question came to the hospital, and, not knowing of this failure in diagnosis, happened to walk through the ward where the child was lying. While walking slowly past the child's bed, but without stopping, he remarked, " That child has pus in his abdomen." This rapid diagnosis was afterwards found to be correct. It is easy to say that this was a lucky guess. But the doctor in question so frequently made lucky guesses of this nature that it was impossible to ascribe them to chance. My informant, who was then at the head of a large hospital, had similar power. He told me that he is sometimes unable to tell the students the reasons for his diagnosis, despite his attempts to call his reasons to mind. The case of another physician has been related to me whose habit of intuitive diagnosis went so far that he was useless as a teacher. Frequently when asked why he had made a particular diagnosis he had to reply, " I am sure I don't know." This power of diagnosis without conscious reasoning seems to be by no means uncommon. Every doctor asked has been able to quote me instances, usually from amongst the staffs of large hospitals who include the picked men of the profession.

In these cases, as in others about to be described, the

act of forgetting is a prelude to the activity in question of the subconscious mind.   If all the facts involved were still present to his consciousness, the doctor would inevitably decide by a process of conscious reasoning. The facts are partly at least forgotten to consciousness and a subconscious diagnosis is made far more rapidly than a decision based on reasoning about remembered facts.

Another example of subconscious judgment is offered by the power that many people possess of rapidly judging character or capacity.   The success of eminent business men, in some cases, appears to depend greatly on their power of rapidly choosing the right man for a particular purpose.   After an acquaintance with a man far too short to admit of any reasoned opinion, their sub-conscious minds give them a verdict as to his capacity on which they rely with confidence.   It is probable that in some cases this power really exists.   But evidence available makes it probable that in other cases, perhaps in the majority of cases, it is little more than a delusion. ⁻ A business man of my acquaintance, who may be referred to as Mr. X, has this power in a remarkable degree and finds it of the greatest use to him in his work.   He sometimes merely concludes that it would be safer not to do business with a particular man.   But sometimes, on the very shortest acquaintance, he feels a strong unreasoning repugnance, which he told me sometimes amounts to a feeling of being paralysed with horror.   For instance, he was once staying in a small village in England.   He went to church and took a dislike of this nature to the clergyman the moment he appeared and before he had begun to speak. Afterwards the clergyman wanted to be introduced to my informant who scandalised his friends by refusing. Some two years afterwards it transpired that the clergyman was a thorough scamp who had defrauded three orphans, to whom he was a guardian. On another occasion an acquaintance wished to introduce Mr. X to a member of a group of religious mystics. Mr. X, having seen this man, promptly refused. Shortly afterwards, in a scandalous police court case, it was shown that this man in question was as unfit as was the late Mr. Squeers for his post as an instructor of youth.

On questioning Mr. X as to the development of this power, very little was found out. He says that, as a child, as often happens with children, he had a habit to taking unreasoning likes and dislikes to people on trivial grounds. At the age of seventeen he went into business. His occupation brought him into contact with fresh people almost every day. He was of a shy disposition and used to listen while others were talking. Occasionally he would feel that a man was peculiar but without being able to decide in what his peculiarity consisted. He would consciously recognise that this vague peculiarity that he had seen in one man was present in another. He told me he would compare them, but what he compared appears to have been the effect the peculiarities produced on him in any two instances. At length he acquired the power of recognising bad characters and people of bad temper. This was all that was necessary to him in his business. He had merely to decide whether or not to trade with any one. He had no need to judge capacity for particular posts and apparently had no special power of doing so. He could recognise a man as being a bad character, he asserted, without hearing his voice and even from a photograph. He can recognise bad character in an Indian but less easily than in an Englishman, but he finds it very difficult to form an opinion of a Chinaman. One singular statement that he made was that a person's reflection in a looking glass was better than a direct view for forming an opinion as to his capacity in the points above mentioned. Mr. X asserts that`he has never made mistakes so long as he has trusted to his first intuitions.

The power of judging character is sometimes strongly developed in women, but no definite evidence is known to me for or against the popular belief that they are endowed with this power more often than men. It is possible that fortune-tellers, so far as what they say is not merely quackery, depend upon subconscious recognition of their clients. A lady fortune-teller told me she depended on intuition and that the palmistry she used was merely a means of humbugging her dupes.

Similar to the power of judging character is the power that some business men claim to possess of estimating the solvency or reliability of people who come to them demanding credit. It is probable that in this case also the power is real in some cases and in other cases is nothing but a delusion.   It is much the same power as that discussed above for it seems to amount to a capacity for judging from a man's demeanour whether he is telling lies about his banking account or his business affairs.

A business man of my acquaintance, who boasts that he has never made a bad debt, has told me of instances in which he has refused credit owing to an intuitive feeling.   In one such instance his friends were angry with him for refusing what appeared to be good business, but which later events proved would have been very bad business indeed.   In such cases there is no doubt that the premonition or intuition is derived from the subconscious mind, for it stands in contradiction to the verdict given by conscious reason.   The applicant for credit perhaps brings with him what appears to reason as unexceptional evidence of his solvency, but nevertheless the business man to whom he makes his application has an intuition to the contrary.   What is to be done ?   In a book called *The Making of a Merchant*, by H. N. Higinbotham, this eventuality is discussed.   The author says that the first time the young merchant " confronts a condition of this kind he may well pause and ask which is the safer guide to follow, intuition or reason.   Speaking from individual experience, I would say, act upon the intuition, for if the case were analysed thoroughly it would be found that the intuition is but the impression gained from a kind of subconscious reasoning."   Here we have a definite statement as to the superiority of subconscious judgment to conscious reason in estimating a man's solvency. The author goes on to give examples which it is needless to quote.

In each of the above instances we are dealing with a mental process of recognition. On receiving certain sensory impressions there is recognition, with the help of the subconscious mind, of a particular disease or a defect of character or of business ability.

It may be suggested that it is very remarkable that the same sensory impressions should produce different effects on the conscious and the subconscious parts of the mind. But such an assertion is unjustified; for there are reasons for believing that the eye, for example, sends to the subconscious mind far more elaborate and detailed impressions than it sends to the conscious mind. The following evidence bears on this point.

In treating of different qualities of wheat, Professor Biffen says : " An experienced buyer can grade wheats with fair accuracy by inspection only, but the grading appears to be dependent on an unconscious recognition of the varieties in question and a previous knowledge of their milling and baking properties." It appears from this statement that different specimens of wheat may have physical differences too small to be consciously noticeable but yet that the eye or the sense of touch may convey knowledge of these differences to the sub-conscious mind, and that this knowledge is used by it in an act of recognition.*

Some years ago when studying the flight of soaring

---

* " Systematised Plant-breeding " in *Science and the Nation* (1st Ed. 1917, Cambridge University Press, p. 168).

birds, by practice my eye became trained to see minute differences in wing adjustments that would be quite invisible to the untrained observer. It seems to me probable that my training was partly connected with my habit of writing down at the time whatever was observed, for it sometimes happened that having seen something, and being aware that it was worth recording and on turning at once to my notebook, I had great difficulty in calling to consciousness exactly what it was that had been seen. About one adjustment that was used for checking speed, it is recorded in my book that though I learnt to recognise when a bird began to use it, there was no change in the appearance of the bird sufficient for me to express in words.* Years afterwards the nature of the adjustment was discovered. It produced a change in outline of the wing-tip that was too small to be recognised by me consciously, but my subconscious mind apparently was aware of the difference and enabled me to know that the bird had changed its mode of flight.†

There are other reasons for thinking that the common term " training one's eye " is inaccurate. The difference between the trained and the untrained observer does not lie in the eye or in the optic nerve. The optic nerve carries the same set of impressions in each case. With the untrained observer fewer of these impressions come through to consciousness than with the trained observer.

These facts do not lead us any nearer to a real explan-

---

* *Animal Flight* (Iliffe and Sons, London, 1913, p. 126).

† See a note " On observation of transiently visible movements " by me in the *Aeronautical Journal*, 1915, p. 104.

ation of subconscious recognition. It may be that more impressions from the eye are available to the sub-conscious mind of a doctor, for example, who makes an almost instantaneous diagnosis for which he is unable to give his reasons, than are available to the conscious mind of another doctor who makes his diagnosis after slow formal reasoning. But if more sensory impressions are available in one case than in the other, how is it that less time is required to deal with them ? This rapidity of action of the subconscious mind, the way in which it appears to deliberate on all the data at once, or nearly at once, is a matter to which we shall revert in a later chapter.

From the point of view of the possibilities of further research, the power of subconscious diagnosis possessed by doctors is more important than the power of estima-ting capacity possessed by business men. From their training doctors are more likely than business men to appreciate a scientific problem and to reply to questions in a way that would satisfy a psychologist. Further, their diagnoses are subject to criticism and control by what happens to the patient. But no such certainty can attach to subconscious acts of recognition by business men. A man of business once described to me how he had been appointed as manager of a jute mill as the result of a five minutes' interview in which no questions were asked as to his capacity and no testimonials had been shown or demanded. My informant made the mill a success. But previously the mill had worked at a loss, and one may well ask whether the previous manager, who was a failure, had not also been appointed after an equally casual interview.

The facts recorded in this chapter indicate that the subconscious mind may exercise, or may be trained to exercise, a power of recognition far higher than the recognition that occurs with the aid of consciousness. In some of the instances quoted—such as grading wheat or my own experiences on the flight of birds—there can be little doubt that the subconscious mind receives and uses sensory impressions too small to affect consciousness. In other instances quoted, such as diagnosis of disease or character, probably the subconscious mind uses impressions of this kind ; but there is room for suspecting that the mental process that occurs is something far more complicated than is involved in recognising that a rose is red.   One suspects that there is a balancing of evidence in the subconscious mind before the diagnosis is made.   In the next chapter examples of the activity of the subconscious mind will be described in which there is yet more reason for suspecting that the decision is arrived at after balancing evidence and after a process of choice.

NOTES

(1) As an illustration of subconscious judgment in estimating character the following incident may be quoted. A medical officer at a certain military hospital in India was impressed by the ability and industry of a subordinate. He thought that this subordinate did not get on as well as he deserved, and hence went out of his way to help him and recommended him for promotion. This medical officer was at length transferred. His successor on the very first occasion that he met the subordinate in question came to the conclusion that he was a scoundrel of the first water. This rapid act of subconscious judgment was very soon proved to be correct, as within a week the subordinate

was arrested for the murder of his wife. He was found guilty of this crime and also of the murder, under atrocious circumstances, of a friend with whose wife he had an intrigue. The case, which was known as the " Clark Murder Case," attracted considerable attention at the time.

(2) Lady Cardigan, in her autobiography, relates how, as a girl, she visited a woman who had a great reputation as a fortune-teller. This woman began by telling her that she would not get married for a long time and that when she did marry she would marry a widower. The woman then went on to foretell various commonplace events that might happen to anybody. The prophecy that she would marry a widower was by no means commonplace. But as the event proved, the fortune-teller had somewhat understated what was to happen. Lady Cardigan says in her singularly frank account :—

" Strangely enough the prediction came true, for Lord Cardigan was a widower, and nearly all the men who proposed to me were widowers. I was asked in marriage by Lord Sherborne, a widower with ten children, by the Duke of Leeds, who was a widower with eleven children, and by Christopher Maunsell Talbot, once Father of the House of Commons, also a widower with four children. Prince Soltykoff, the Duke of St. Albans, Harry Howard, and Disraeli, were other widowers who proposed to me, so I suppose I must have had some unaccountable fascination for bereaved husbands."*

Whether or not the fortune-teller had had experience that girls who marry later rather than sooner are more attractive to men of mature experience and age, and recognised that the future Lady Cardigan was of a disposition to hesitate before entering the marriage state, it is a fact that different classes of women are attractive to different classes of men. It would not be very wonderful if the fortune-teller had subconsciously recognised to which class Lady Cardigan belonged and so was able, to some small extent, to predict her future.

---

* *My Recollections*, by the Countess of Cardigan (George Bell and Sons, London, 1909), p. 38.

CHAPTER III

EXAMPLES OF SUBCONSCIOUS JUDGMENT

The instinctive mental powers of statesmen and administrators
—The jury system as an example of the use of subconscious
judgment—Recently acquired knowledge bad for such
judgment—The value of forgetting—Comparison of committees and juries—Lord Mansfield's advice never to give
reasons—Cross examination—-Rapid composition by journalists—Sherlock Holmes in practice.

We will now consider other examples of subconscious
judgment that appear to be of a higher order of com-
plexity than those hitherto discussed. Their nature is
such as to suggest that processes analogous to choice
and formal reason may go on in the subconscious mind
of a higher degree of efficiency than occur in the region
of consciousness.

An important instance is the instinctive power of
rapid decision possessed by statesmen and administrators. Of Lord Kitchener it is recorded that " he had a
most extraordinary instinct in military matters. He
never thought things out. He seemed to know them."
Here the power of rapid decision was not due to formal
reason but to its replacement by work of the subconscious mind, the result of which alone came into his
consciousness.

Mr. J. M. Keynes thus describes Mr. Lloyd George's
activities at the Peace Conference :—

" What chance could such a man [President Wilson]

have against Mr. Lloyd George's unerring, almost medium-like sensibility to every one immediately around him ?   To see the British Prime Minister watching the company, with six or seven senses not available to ordinary men, judging character, motive, and subconscious impulse, perceiving what each was thinking and even what each was going to say next, and compounding with telepathic instinct the argument or appeal best suited to the vanity, weakness, or self-interest of his immediate auditor, was to realise that the poor President would be playing blind man's buff in such a party."*

Such instinctive mental powers of Mr. Lloyd George are not due to an abnormal amount or even perhaps to a normal amount of knowledge.   Here are other opinions of him : " M. Clemenceau exclaimed of him, lifting up amazed hands, ' I have never met so ignorant a man as Lloyd George ! '   A greater wit said of him, ' I believe Mr. Lloyd George *can* read, but I am perfectly certain he never does.' "†

As an example of the prevalent belief that instinct is more important than formal reason to a statesman, the following opinion expressed by Mr. F. S. Oliver may be quoted :

" Looked at from the strictly intellectual standpoint, the reasons which satisfied German statesmen with

---

* *The Economic Consequences of the Peace* (London, Macmillan and Co., 1920), p. 37.

† From *The Mirrors of Downing Street*, by " A Gentleman with a Duster " (London, Mills and Boon, 1920).

regard to Britain's neutrality were overwhelming, and might well have convinced others, of a similar outlook and training, who had no personal interest whatsoever in coming to one conclusion rather than another.

" None the less the judgment of the Kaiser and his Ministers was not only bad, but inexcusably bad. We expect more from statesmen than that they should arrive at logical conclusions. Logic in such cases is nothing ; all that matters is to be right ; but unless instinct rules and reason serves, right judgment will rarely be arrived at in such matters as these. If a man cannot feel as well as reason, if he cannot gauge the forces which are at work among the nations by some kind of second sight, he has no title to set up his bills as a statesman."*

Thus the decisions of statesmen and administrative officials differ from those of formal reasoning in that they are largely influenced by results of experience that do not enter consciousness. They are also often characterised by the extreme rapidity with which they are reached. An expert dealing with an affair of test-tubes may take weeks or months before he is satisfied that his data are sufficient for a reasoned decision. Our fellow men are far more complicated than test-tubes. Nevertheless administrators, statesmen and men of business often decide about them with great rapidity and in the absence of sufficient data for the employment of formal reason. If such reason were the only mental weapon of the statesman he would require far more

* *Ordeal by Battle*, p. 68.

time for a decision than does an expert when dealing with his test-tubes. The statesman necessarily relies on the intuitive power of his mind. However useful this power may be, it has a defect that forms one of the most serious of our mental limitations. As we shall see in Chapter V., such intuitive power depends, in some complicated way, on our past experiences. If the past experiences of a statesman have been only with men of his own race and his own mode of thinking, it is only with such men that his intuitions will be reliable. Here we have the psychological justification for the saying that it is necessary to trust the man on the spot. The man on the spot, at least if he has been there a long time, will have intuitions based on his experiences there obtained. However unconvincing his reasons may be, his intuitive judgment is likely to be better than that of the statesman at home. The judgment of the Kaiser and his Ministers would probably have been valid if they had had to deal only with men of German temperament. It is a historical fact that their judgment ran counter to the advice of eminent German diplomatists who had gained their experience abroad. The German advisers of the Kaiser failed to trust the man on the spot with highly unfortunate results.

The out-of-place politician, on the other hand, demands from his subconscious mind not only conclusions but also facts on which such conclusions are based, for it is his business to discover and ventilate grievances the remedying of which will, if possible, discredit government.

The statesman and the administrative official would be hard put to it if they had to tackle every problem that comes before them by the scientific methods of Sherlock Holmes. The interest that the character of Sherlock Holmes arouses is in great part due to the fact that, in real life, it so rarely happens that we are able to rely on formal reason alone for any but the most straightforward problems. When, in fiction, we read of this happening, the singularity of the occurrence at once fixes our attention and our curiosity.

An illustration of the power of subconscious judgment possessed by ordinary people is to be found in the success of the jury system.

A jury consists of men probably ignorant of law, probably unaccustomed to hearing and interpreting evidence, probably lacking the mental agility of barristers in appreciating a new subject and probably destitute of scientific training ; yet there is a consensus of opinion among legal authorities that in judging of matters of fact they often give better verdicts than the judges themselves.

It may be thought that a jury having listened to the reasoned arguments of counsel and the reasoned summing up of the judge, and having heard the evidence of witnesses on which the reasoning in the case is based, must necessarily use their conscious reason in coming to a verdict.

It would be difficult for me to counter this view were it not for my own experience on juries. On the first occasion, despite careful attention, my success in remembering the evidence was very partial. It was soon obvious to me that my recollections were being driven out of my consciousness by the effect of their quantity. There were speeches for the prosecution, speeches for the defence, evidence on one side and the other, cross-examinations, and then, after the partial speeches of the counsel, the very impartial summing up of the judge. It is a usual experience that if one tries to remember too much at once one forgets everything. If one hears a good joke or a good story one may remember it, but if one hears twenty jokes or twenty good stories at a sitting, one forgets them all. In this case too much evidence and too much argument had been administered and my feeling was that none of the important evidence had remained in my consciousness. In such circumstances it was highly embarassing to have to come to a decision, for not only was the evidence forgotten, but what was remembered was the difficulty I had had in appreciating its import. My fellow jurymen, however, had no such embarassment. There were no grounds for suspecting that their recollection of the evidence was better than mine. But they were quite contented. They were practical men, and, as such, were not accustomed to the formal arguments that are habitual with the expert. The fact that they had forgotten the details of the evidence meant that these details had been driven from consciousness to the subconscious mind. The conclusion is unavoidable that these details because they were in the subconscious mind were available to it in forming a decision which was then pushed forward into consciousness. The members of the jury came at once to an unanimous conclusion that the prisoner was guilty. They did so, relying on common sense and not on any attempt at adequate formal reasoning. On the second occasion of my serving on a jury, profiting by my previous experience, and being then aware of the value of forgetting, I made no effort to remember the evidence and found no more difficulty than did the other jurymen in forming an opinion.

The authority, from whom the opinions of lawyers on the jury system are about to be quoted, remarks that " Juries are generally right, more often indeed than judges and counsel, because they judge from a common-sense point of view." The judge and the counsel having a better power of appreciating and remembering the evidence of the jury, have it at their fingers' ends. So long as this is the case they are confined to those reasoned decisions that in the complicated affairs of life and when dealing with our fellow men are often of less value than those judgments in which our subconscious minds play the larger part. The judge and the counsel use formal reason and can only use such reason because the facts of the case are present to their consciousness. The jury have, for the most part, forgotten the facts. They therefore give a common-sense verdict by an action of the subconscious mind. If delay occurs before they agree on their verdict, it is occupied in reasoning in which the facts are very imperfectly remembered and which reasoning is subordinated to the intuitive feelings of the majority. " Sometimes," said Sir Archibald

Smith, " I think the verdict of the jury is wrong and I feel disappointed in it, but I think the case over, and I find on reflection that the jury were quite right." Thus, to one who necessarily uses formal reasoning at the outset, "second thoughts are best" because delay allows the evidence to be less strongly impressed on his conscious mind and therefore to be the more available to take part in an act of subconscious judgment.

The judge and counsel, at the time, must have their minds dominated by their knowledge of the case, both because it has been recently acquired and because it has been acquired as the result of their own knowledge and research. That knowledge thus acquired is inimical to duly balanced judgment will be shown when we come to consider the mental limitations of the globe-trotter. Further evidence is found in the common advice to sleep over a thing before deciding. Such advice is only given and is only appropriate when an act of judgment is required on recently acquired knowledge in which one happens to be interested. One's interest in the matter by keeping the facts within reach of consciousness, keeps them away from the purview of the subconscious mind ; we are therefore in a position to treat them by means of our conscious reason but not with the added help of our subconscious judgment. After a change in the current of our thoughts and a night's sleep, when the facts in question are no longer so vividly present to our consciousness, we are in a position to use the subconscious mind besides our conscious reason in coming to a decision.

D

A corollary from the above explanation of the value of juries is that one would not expect professional or expert jurymen to be a success. They would develop a habit of remembering too much of what they had heard. They would be liable to be overimpressed by some details of the evidence ; this they would use in formal arguments instead of arriving at common-sense verdicts.

Another corollary is that the success of the jury system in England and America is not by itself a proof that it would be a success with other nationalities. Indians, for instance, often have far better memories than Englishmen. Hence it is possible that a jury of Indians would use, or tend to use, formal argument rather than subconscious judgment. Lombroso has strongly criticised the jury system in Italy.* He admits that it is a success with Anglo-Saxons but asserts that, in Italy, jurymen are too often influenced by matters outside the evidence they have heard. But Lombroso's arguments seem to be of a somewhat *a priori* nature and it would be advisable, before accepting his views, to learn the opinion of Italian legal authorities on the subject.

It will be worth while to devote a little more discussion to the jury system. In the first place, the suggestion that its value is that it elicits the average opinion of twelve men will not hold water. A jury does not give " average " verdicts. It gives extreme verdicts— " guilty " or " not guilty."

---

* *Crime and its remedies*, 1911, p. 353.

Secondly, as regards comparing a jury with a committee, it is widely different from the kind of committee known as a Royal Commission. For a committee of this kind persons eminent in different branches of the subject are carefully selected. They can and do use their formal reasoning powers, as they have time and capacity for this method of mental activity. Months or years may elapse before they agree on their report. They are not expected to arrive at an immediate conclusion as is a jury.

Neither is it fair to compare a jury with a committee formed by the heads of separate government departments who confer together on some administrative point. Here the members are all men of administrative experience who are accustomed to serve on such committees. Committees of this nature have stood the test of experience.

The members of a jury are men chosen at haphazard, men presumably ignorant of law and unaccustomed to balance legal evidence. The kind of committee to which a jury may fairly be compared is one chosen in a haphazard way, such as a club committee. However successful such committees may be in dealing with permanent interests or routine work, there are good grounds for asserting that they are unsatisfactory for dealing with some special point or emergency. It is then found that one man talks without being able to decide ; another decides without listening to argument ; arguments fail to retain their proper relative importance. For any or all of these reasons it often happens that evidence is not fairly considered and that the man who talks loudest carries the day. Similarly it has been said by Macaulay that no army commanded by a debating society was ever led to victory.

Reference has been made to the opinions of eminent legal authorities on the subject of juries. None of them complain that the man with the longest tongue has an undue influence. None of them say that a man on a jury is not at his best. On the contrary they find that a jury is the best means of arriving at a rapid conclusion on a matter of fact. If it were merely a question of getting an average opinion of twelve men a committee ought to be even more successful than a jury. But it is not. The difference lies in the fact that in a law court there is a division of labour. Some, the witnesses, bring forward evidence. Others, the counsel, discuss it. The judge sums up ; while the jury only listens and gives the verdict. On a committee each member acts, or may act, both as witness, as advocate, as judge and as jury. The members of a committee themselves bring forward the evidence, or perhaps are previously acquainted with it. It is present to their consciousness. They remember it and therefore can only use it in reasoned arguments. The members of the jury do not produce evidence by their own exertion. There is nothing, therefore, to impress it on their consciousness. It is flung at them in such quantities that their consciousness can only retain a vague general idea of its nature. What they have forgotten is at the disposal of their subconscious minds. They therefore arrive at a verdict by an act of subconscious judgment, As with previous instances quoted the forgetting of the facts is a prelude to the activity of the subconscious mind.

The practice of appointing persons who are not administrators to the heads of administrations may be explained and defended in the same way as the jury system. A functionary holding such a post knows but little of administrative details. The reasoned views on any point in the government of a Crown Colony, for example, are put before him together with the comments of the permanent officials of the office. If he is a normal individual it is almost impossible for him to reason adequately on the subject. The details are too many to all remain in consciousness. He therefore is obliged to employ his subconscious judgment. The comments of the permanent officials correspond to the summing up of the judge, while he himself represents the jurymen who give the common-sense verdict. *A priori* one would expect that difficulties might arise if the individual appointed to such a post was a man whose memory and power of conscious reasoning was abnormally developed. Many years ago, an Indian gentleman, who was well-disposed towards the government of India, wrote a letter to a newspaper in which he said that the diplomatic type of Englishman was not suitable for governing. " For," said he, " if an Englishman is a clever diplomat, we Indians can twist him round our little finger." Apparently, to quote the " original German," he shared the opinion of Heine to the effect that " Gegen den Dumheit kämpfen die Götte vergebenst."*

The importance of subconscious judgment, though under other names, has long been recognised. In describing the reform of the currency in the reign of William III, Macaulay refers to two philosophers who helped in deciding what was to be done, as men " in whom habits of abstruse meditation had not impaired that homely good sense without which even genius is mischievous in politics." The philosophers discussed the problem with two politicians and Macaulay says : " It would be interesting to see how the pure gold of scientific truth found by the two philosophers was mingled by the two statesmen with just that quantity of alloy which was necessary for the working." Evidently the alloy here referred to is what has been described as the power of subconscious judgment.

The following story, told of Lord Mansfield, well illustrates the superiority, in certain cases, of subconscious judgment over formal reasoning.

First it may be explained that Lord Mansfield (1705-1793) was one of the greatest of English lawyers and is regarded as the founder of English mercantile law. It happened that a friend of his was appointed Governor of a West Indian Island. He told Lord Mansfield that the one thing he dreaded about his post was that he would have to sit as a judge and decide cases. Upon which Lord Mansfield advised him to decide according to his notions of commonsense, but

---

* Against stupidity, the Gods fight in vain.

never to give his reasons ; " for," said he, " your judgments will probably be right, but your reasons will certainly be wrong."

Thus one of the greatest of English lawyers, whose profound knowledge of the law and whose long experience enabled him to rely on his formal reason, advised his friend, who had no experience, to mistrust his formal reason and imitate the jury in relying, in legal matters, on his subconscious judgment.

There was a curious sequel to the story. Some years afterwards, Lord Mansfield, while sitting on Privy Council appeals, had a judgment of this Governor brought before his court, which seemed so absurd in its reasons that there was serious clamour for the recall of the Governor as incompetent. It was found, however, that the decision itself was perfectly right. It appeared that, at first, the Governor had acted on Lord Mansfield's advice by deciding without giving reasons ; and, finding that he acquired a great reputation thereby, began to think himself a great lawyer, and then, at length, took to giving his reasons with the above-mentioned result.*

We next come to an example of a mental activity about which there is room for doubt how far it is due to conscious reasoning and how far to subconscious judgment. Every barrister is aware that in cross-examination, especially in criminal cases, it is important to know when to stop. If one does not stop at the right point evidence may be elicited that helps the opposite

---

* Croake James, *Curiosities of Law and Lawyers* (Sampson Law, London, 1882), p. 59.

side instead of one's own.   Experienced barristers can stop but inexperienced barristers sometimes cannot stop at the right point.   The barrister has to make up his mind when to stop on the spur of the moment. Generally it is the answer that he has just received, perhaps an unexpected answer, that determines him to finish his questioning.   Barristers can sometimes reason very quickly.   They may be conscious of their reasons for stopping but there is at least a possibility that their reasons are known only to their subconscious minds.

An interesting example of a developed habit of being aided by subconscious judgment is offered by the journalist who rapidly writes a brilliant descriptive article on the spur of first impressions.   This facile writing of the journalist may be contrasted with the method perforce employed by the expert.   In an article giving advice to young experts on composition the recommendation is given that they should use a large waste-paper basket. On any point several possible methods of arranging his data will occur to the expert.   He has to make a choice by a slow and laborious exercise of his conscious reason.   In my own experience, so frequently is the least objectionable method the last to appear, and so much better is it than the others, as to suggest that the subconscious mind is reluctant to part with the idea that pleases it most.   Possibly we have here a clue to Lord Mansfield's dictum that though your judgments may be right " your reasons will certainly be wrong." The journalist probably only thinks of one method of expressing himself, or, if other ideas do occur to him, they make no strong impression and he has no difficulty in discarding them. Probably everyone who has composed will agree that sometimes he can write rapidly, as does the journalist, and sometimes slowly, as does the expert, and that he has experienced every intermediate degree of facility in composing.

The most plausible explanation of these differing modes of composition is that numerous ideas occur alike to the journalist and to the expert, but that only in the case of the expert do they all come through from the subconscious mind into consciousness. It may be suggested that the subconscious mind of the journalist is so constituted that it exercises choice and sends on to consciousness only the chosen mode of expression. Hence his conscious reason has little or no occasion to hesitate between alternatives. If this explanation is correct, one would expect that much practice in exercise in formal reasoning, though useful to the scholar and to the expert, might be detrimental to the journalist. As evidence pointing in this direction the following opinions may be quoted. Mr. G. Ranger Gull says :—

" In popular and semi-popular journalism, the University man is nearly always a failure. He has not the faculty of feeling the public pulse. He imagines his judgments are literary when they are merely narrow."*

Mr. Kennedy Jones has expressed the following opinion :—

" But for a recorder or reporter of news the first

* *Back to Lilac Land*, p. 185.

essential is the news instinct.   It is a natural gift and is rarer than is commonly supposed.   I doubt if not being born in a man it is ever acquired.   It is certainly something apart from education.   Send to any common-place event, such as a wedding or a funeral, an Oxford honours graduate deficient in the news instinct, and a Board School youth endowed with it, and the former will hand in a report, written perhaps in perfect prose, accurate in detail, but dull as ditchwater, while the other, in common colloquial English, will depict the very scene, and by his instinctive choice of essentials and of the broad humanities, though they may appear superficially trivial, convey to the reader the very scene itself, as though he were witness to it "*

NOTES.

(1) Sir William Robertson expressed himself about Lord Kitchener as follows : Kitchener had· a most extraordinary instinct in military matters. He never thought things out. He seemed to know them. This faculty of his amounted to genius. People who criticise him for his mistakes forget that he was seldom wrong in the big things. Some infallible instinct guided him in matters of life and death."† Contemporary criticisms of Lord Kitchener dealt almost entirely with matters in which formal reason was required rather than subconscious judgment.

(2) a.   As an illustration of the methods of Sherlock Holmes being used in real life, the following story told of the late Sir Astley Cooper may be quoted.   A man sitting in a hotel at Rotherhithe was murdered by someone who opened the door of the room where his victim was sitting and shot him dead with a pistol.   From the position of the body, the position of the wound, and the position of the door, Sir Astley Cooper deduced that the man who fired the shot must have been left-handed.   A man named Patch was arrested on suspicion.   He

---

* *Fleet Street and Downing Street* (Hutchinson & Co., London, 1919), p. 29.

† An interview published in the *New York Times*.

denied that he was left-handed. At that time it was customary for an accused to hold up his hand when pleading guilty or not guilty. Patch, unfortunately for him, held up his left hand. He was convicted and executed.

(2) b. A box of calcined bones was sent to me and I was requested to report whether they were the remains of a man or a woman. No fragment of the bones was more than two inches long. A piece of green glass was noticed attached to one of the fragments. It was of the same colour as the glass commonly used in India for women's bangles. In my report it was suggested that this fact indicated that the bones were of a female, if, in the district from which they came, glass bangles were worn by women and not by men.

(2) c. It is obvious that the above two instances are of an exceptional nature and are far from proving that the methods of Sherlock Holmes could be used by any finite intelligence in most of the affairs of life. The following instance of a failure in applying such methods resembles far more what is likely to happen in practice. An elderly lady had died at Mussoorie, an Indian hill station, under circumstances that suggested poisoning. Prussic acid was detected in the portion of her viscera that was sent me for examination. There was no evidence as to how this poison had been administered. Among other articles sent for examination were the ashes from the grate in the lady's bedroom. In them was found a veronal tabloid. It was seen by me that it was slightly thicker than a tabloid from a bottle of such tabloids that had been found in her bedroom. The difference in thickness was about half a millimetre. On putting one of these tabloids into my mouth, spitting it out after a few seconds and keeping it for some hours, it was found to have swelled up and to be of exactly the same thickness as the tabloid from the ashes. The obvious inference was that the lady had put a tabloid into her mouth before going to bed, had felt the symptoms of prussic acid poisoning coming on and had, therefore, spat out the tabloid, got into bed and died. Hence the observation suggested that it was a case of murder and not suicide. Fortunately my report dealt only with the facts, as it afterwards transpired that a doctor, who came into the room after the death was discovered, had found the bottle of veronal tabloids, had taken one out, bitten off a small piece and then spat out the remainder into the fireplace. It had been noticed by me that a very small piece of the tabloid was missing. It appeared to me to be probable that this had been broken off by the tabloid having hit the firebars or the back of the fireplace when it was spat out. Sherlock Holmes, no doubt, would have had in his mind a complete knowledge of the fragility of veronal tabloids before and after being sucked and of their velocities

when ejected into fireplaces by aged ladies and young doctors respectively and thus would have been able to deduce the history of the tabloid.   Obviously it is far from feasible for a detective to have his head as full of detailed knowledge of an infinity of trivial matters as would be necessary were he to rely solely on the methods of Sherlock Holmes in every case that came in his way.

(3) a.   " As a rule," said Sir Edward Carson, K.C., when interviewed on the subject, " juries return good verdicts.   I should prefer a jury's verdict to that of a judge, and I think it is a great pity that judges should interfere so much with the free exercise of their opinion by juries ; in many instances, indeed, usurping their functions, for the juries naturally don't like to set up views against the experience of a trained judge."

(3) b.   " A jury assisted by a judge is a far better tribunal for the elucidation of the truth than a judge unassisted by a jury," observed Sir Alexander Cockburn.

(3) c.   " A jury is, in general, far more likely to come to a right decision than a judge," remarked Chief Justice Erle.   " As a rule juries are, in my opinion, more right than judges."

(3) d.   Some years ago Lord Halsbury, addressing the United Law Society, said : " For myself, I will avow that trial by jury is too often lightly regarded, and that it is one of the surest foundations on which civil rights repose.   As a rule, juries are, in my opinion, more generally right than judges."

(3) e.   The late Lord Russell of Killowen held a very strong opinion on the value of a jury as judges of matters of fact.   He always thought that the average opinion of twelve men of common sense was at least equal to the judgment of twelve judges on matters of fact.

The above opinions on the value of juries are from a book by Mr. H. E. Fenn, called, *Thirty-five years in the Divorce Court.*

(3) f.   Mr. Sergeant Ballantine says : " During my experience I have rarely known a thoroughly innocent person convicted, although there are certain charges scarcely sustained by strict evidence, but which carry with them a moral conclusion, and in which juries are apt to reject law and yield to prejudice ; but little evil arises from such results, and substantial justice is obtained.   I must, however, except one class of case in which I have seen very grave errors committed by juries, and I fear many innocent people have suffered.   I allude to charges preferred by women against the opposite sex.   Juries in many of these instances seem to bid adieu to common sense.   The tears

of a good-looking girl efface arguments of counsel and the suggestions of reason. However absurd and incredible the story told may be, a fainting fit at an appropriate time removes from their minds all its improbabilities. I have often wished that such charges might be disposed of by a jury of matrons."*

(4) a. The following story, told me by the late Sir George Paget, is a striking example of a barrister not knowing when to stop his cross-examination. A man named Thurtell, a gambler, was indicted for the murder of someone who he wished to rob at some time early in the nineteenth century. A junior counsel for the defence was cross-examining a barmaid at an hotel that Thurtell was supposed to have visited at the time. It was vital for the prosecution to prove that Thurtell had done so. The barmaid recognised the man in the dock as having come into the bar on the day in question though, as she admitted, she had only seen him, outside the dock, on this single occasion. " How many visitors do you have in your bar every day ? " asked the counsel. " Between a hundred and fifty and two hundred," replied the witness. The senior barrister for the defence at once, by a gesture, attempted to hint to his colleague that he should ask no more questions. Unfortunately for the prisoner the hint was not taken. " How can you expect me to believe that you can remember one particular man," enquired the counsel, out of a couple of hundred that come daily into your bar ? " " When I saw him," replied the barmaid, " I thought him the most good-looking man I had ever seen." The jury looked at Thurtell and saw that he was good-looking. This sealed his fate. He was convicted and executed.

(4) b. The following is an instance of a barrister knowing when to stop his cross-examination. A woman was under trial for poisoning her husband. She was defended by Ballantine who suspected that she was guilty. The following is taken from his account : " It is sufficient to say that a minute quantity of arsenic was discovered in the body of the deceased, which in the defence I accounted for by the suggestion that poison had been used carelessly for the destruction of rats. Mr. Baron Parke summed up not unfavourably to the prisoner, dwelling pointedly upon the small quantity of arsenic found in the body, and the jury without much hesitation acquitted her. . . . Dr. Taylor the professor of chemistry, and an experienced witness, had proved the presence of arsenic, and, as I imagine, to the great disappointment of my solicitor, who desired a severe cross-examination, I did not ask him a single question. He was sitting

---

* *Some Experiences of a Barrister's Life*, by Mr. Sergeant Ballantine, p. 103.

on the bench and near the judge, who, after he had summed up and before the verdict was pronounced, remarked to him that he was surprised at the small amount of arsenic found; upon which, Taylor said that if he had been asked the question he should have proved that it indicated, under the circumstances detailed in evidence, that a very large quantity had been taken. The professor had learnt never to volunteer evidence, and the counsel for the prosecution had omitted to put the necessary question. Mr. Baron Parke having learnt the circumstance by accidental means, did not feel warranted in using the information and I had my first lesson in the art of " silent cross-examination."*

---

* Ballantine, *loc. cit.*, p. 161.

CHAPTER IV

ON ABNORMAL CALCULATING POWER

Comparison of common sense and rapid calculating power—Calculators of defective intelligence—Calculators of high general ability—Recognising numbers at a glance—Memory for figures—Bidder's methods—Colburn's methods—Memory experts—Several processes occurring simultaneously as explanation of rapid calculating.

If one says to a business man, and if the idea is new to him, that being rich doesn't consist in having money : it consists in having more money than other people— he instantly smiles. But on making this remark to a socialist, he was observed by me to frown instantly. In either case a moment's thought was all that was needed to form an opinion. But what a number of past experiences, of stored data, of preconceived ideas, of beliefs and feelings, must be involved and must be used by the subconscious mind to produce the smile or the frown ! And what time would be needed to bring them all out into consciousness and to weigh them in conscious reasoning ! It is this extreme rapidity of the work of the subconscious mind that is its salient character and that most urgently needs to be explained.

The instances of the mental activity of the subconscious mind dealt with in the preceding chapters have thrown no light on this point. The examples chosen have been commonplace and typical. Now it

is well recognised that, if we wish to describe a phenomenon, it is necessary to take typical examples, but if
we wish to explain a phenomenon it is advisable to
consider exceptions. An exceptional instance is offered
by cases of abnormal calculating power. The speed at
which lightning calculators produce their results may
be compared to the speed with which we arrive at a
common-sense decision. If we can explain this speed
in one case, we may hope to have some clue to its nature
in the other.

In the year 1813, Zerah Colburn, a boy of nine years,
gave demonstrations in London of his remarkable
powers of rapid calculation. He could do in his head
long sums of multiplication and division and extract
square and cube roots, though he was stated to be
"entirely ignorant of the commonest rules of arithmetic." He usually gave his answers as fast as the
questions could be written down. On one occasion
"the person appointed to take down the results was
obliged to enjoin him not to be so rapid." Further, if
he was given such a number as 171,395, he would
instantly say that it was equal to 5 × 34,279. It was
equal, he said, to

$$7 \times 24,415$$
$$59 \times 2,905$$
$$83 \times 2,065$$
$$35 \times 4,897$$
$$295 \times 581$$
$$\text{and} \quad 413 \times 415$$

These pairs of numbers are called "factors" of the

number 171,395. Thus Colburn differed from most persons of abnormal calculating power in having a remarkable intuitive power of "factorising." This power, as we shall see, is a matter of great psychological interest.

Of another calculator, G. P. Bidder, it is related that "Two days before his death (aged 72), the query was suggested that taking the velocity of light at 190,000 miles per second, and the wave length of the red rays at 36,918 to an inch, how many of its waves must strike the eye in one second? His friend, producing a pencil, was about to calculate the result, when Mr. Bidder said, " You need not work it : the number of vibrations will be four hundred and forty-four billions, four hundred and thirty-three thousand six hundred and fifty-one millions, two hundred thousand vibrations." This number written in figures is 444,433,651,200,000.

We shall get some help in discussing such feats of calculation by using a simile that my brother, Mr. G. T. Hankin, H.M.I., of the Education Department, tells me he employs in explaining the process of dealing with new impressions. The mind, he says, is like a government office. Letters brought by the postman (our sensory impressions) are first opened by junior clerks and attached to their appropriate files. That is to say sense impressions are first associated with previously received impressions that are related to them. The files are then sent up to the senior clerks who compare them with other files which they send for from the " registry " (the reasoned memory). On these data

E

they make notes, either as tentative decisions which are then sent to the director's office, or, choosing between the tentative decisions, they make a final decision which alone is submitted to the director. The latter takes necessary action, marks the files " DW " (done with) and sends them away to be stored by the senior clerks until they are needed for making another decision.

We will use this simile in describing abnormal calculating ability. With persons having this power, it is obvious that, in terms of our simile, the department dealing with figures is overstaffed. As to how this happens, two possibilities suggest themselves. Either the over-staffing is attained by robbing other departments or it may be due to a congenital excessive number of clerks. We shall see that abnormal calculators fall into two classes in accordance with these anticipations.

First, if abnormal calculating power is due to robbing other departments, we may expect that, in such cases, there will be defects of intelligence. The following are examples :

The calculator Dase was described as being of extreme stupidity. Despite his remarkable powers, " it was impossible to get him to comprehend the first beginning of mathematics."

Wizel relates a case of a woman of considerable calculating power who is in an imbecile condition. Her power of judgment is on the level of that of a child of three years.

Elliott mentions a half idiot who was remarkable for his powers of calculation.

Jedediah Buxton had "not even ordinary intelligence in ordinary matters of life." Owing to excessive stupidity when a child he had had no education except that he learnt the multiplication table. Outside arithmetic he retained fewer ideas than a boy of ten years. When taken to a theatre to see Garrick act he attended to him only to count the number of words he uttered.

Zerah Colburn was a very backward child and of mediocre intelligence in adult life.

Mondeux could not remember a name or an address. His intelligence was below the average though a committee reported that "he invents processes, sometimes remarkable, to solve various questions which are ordinarily treated with the aid of algebra."

Inaudi had a bad memory for daily trivial affairs. He could not learn historical dates. He was very ignorant and lacking in intellectual needs.

If such defects of intelligence as the above are due (following our simile) to abnormal transfer of clerks, we may anticipate that on a sufficient stimulus they might be sent back to their proper departments. Facts in agreement with this expectation are as follows :

In 1814, when in Paris, the public performances of Colburn were interrupted for three months while he was learning French with the result that "even in this short space it was observable that he had lost in the quickness of his computations." Before long his power of rapid calculation left him completely.

Archbishop Whately of Dublin had a calculating faculty which began at an age between 5 and 6 and lasted for about three years. He says : " When I went to school, at which time the passion wore off, I was a perfect dunce at ciphering and have continued so ever since."

Mangiamele, Mondeux, Prolongeau, Safford and Mr. Van R of Utica are other calculators whose power only lasted a few years.

Thus in the above instances the abnormal calculating power was due to a mental defect. This conclusion is not without a practical bearing. If a boy shows special aptitude in some particular subject, then, before encouraging him to specialise in it, it is advisable to be sure that his aptitude is not due to robbing other departments.

In the above class of cases in which abnormal calculating power is of the nature of a mental defect, physical or other defects are also sometimes present. Colburn had supernumerary toes. Mondeux was hysterical. Grandmange was born without arms or legs. Colburn in his memoir mentions a calculator who showed symptoms resembling St. Vitus's dance so long as he was doing a calculation. Fleury was born blind and was " of inferior general mentality if not actually insane."

The other alternative possibility is that the calculating power is due to a congenital surplus number of clerks. In such cases we may expect that the surplus will also exist in other departments, besides in that dealing with figures, with resulting general ability above the normal. The following instances are to the point :

Ampère had calculating ability. He became a distinguished mathematician.   He learnt an encyclopædia by heart and fifty years later could repeat long passages of it accurately.

Gauss showed calculating ability at the age of 14. He learnt classics with great ease and had a successful career as a mathematician.

Bidder, the best known of the English calculators, became an engineer and was " of first-rate business ability and of rapid and clear insight into what would pay."

His son G. Bidder Q.C. also had calculating power. At the university he was 7th wrangler.   He afterwards became a barrister of repute.

Safford showed calculating power at the age of six. After he had lost the power of rapid calculation, he continued to take pleasure in factoring large numbers or in satisfying himself that they were prime.   He became a professor of astronomy.

It is of interest to notice that it is only in this class of calculators in which, to continue the simile, we are dealing with a surplus of clerks and not a robbing of other departments that there is any evidence of heredity influence.

For instance, George Parker Bidder was the son of an English stone mason.   A brother was an excellent mathematician.   An elder brother had an unusually good memory and an inclination for figures but could not calculate.   A nephew had mechanical ingenuity. His son George Bidder Q.C. inherited his talent.   The two daughters of this son had calculating powers above the average. A granddaughter had great visual memory.

Diamandi, a Greek, when at school was always first in mathematics. He learnt five languages. When grown up he wrote verses and stories. One sister and one brother were good at calculating.

Before trying to discover the nature of abnormal calculating power, it will be well to consider some mental powers that are not the sole and essential part of this ability.

First, there is the power of rapidly recognising numbers. The calculator Dase needed only a glance to tell him the number of a flock of sheep or the number of a handful of peas (up to about thirty in number) thrown on the ground or the number of letters in a line of print. This power is not recorded for other calculators and it is met with in persons who have no calculating ability. A Spanish-American conjuror told me he had the power of instantly estimating the number of his audience, which power was of use to him when attempts were made to cheat him of his gate money. In an Indian gambling game a handful of cowries is thrown down. The spectators often have a remarkable power of instantly knowing how many will be left over if the cowries are counted off in groups of four. Houdin, the celebrated French conjuror, if he passed a toyshop, could carry away an impression of the numbers and kinds of each different article he had seen in the window. He taught himself to do this by learning to recognise instantly the total number of points on a number of dominoes. On seeing a group of dominoes his subconscious mind, counted the points and the total alone was sent up to consciousness. Similarly Scripture taught himself on seeing any two single figure numbers written, to know their total at a glance before he consciously recognised the value of each individual number. As will be mentioned below the calculator Diamandi seems to have been slow in recognising the import of a row of numbers.

Secondly, calculators often have a remarkable memory for figures but there is no evidence that the best calculators have the best memory but rather the reverse. Jedediah Buxton had the most remarkable memory of all but was the slowest and least clever at calculating. Bidder, on the contrary, the most capable perhaps of recorded calculators, had a limited figure memory. In explaining why, in multiplying, he began at the left hand end of a row of figures, he says, " I could neither remember the figures (in the ordinary way of multiplying) nor could I, unless by a great effort, on a particular occasion, recollect a series of lines of figures."

The case of Jedediah Buxton is worth our attention in this respect. It is recorded of him that " So retentive is his memory, that he will repeat his answers a month or two afterwards if you ask him." He could give the figures of an answer, which might be thirty or more digits, either backwards or forwards. " He will leave a long question half wrought and at the end of several months resume it beginning where he left off." He appears to have done very little thinking about the figures that he stored so exactly in his memory. For instance, in order to multiply a number by 100, he first multiplied it by 5 and then by 20. He had actually failed to discover that a hundred times a number can be got simply by adding to it 00.

Buxton's calculations were slow. It seems to have been a frequent practice with him to commence when he woke up in the morning at the point where he left off at night. Such a fact suggests that his computing was a conscious process, but it is stated that " He will talk with you freely while doing his questions, it being no molestation to him, but enough to confound a penman." Similarly Binet remarks with regard to the calculator Inaudi : " We have seen him sustain a conversation with M. Charcot at the Salpetriere while he solved mentally a complicated problem ; this conversation did not confuse him in his calculations, it simply prolonged their duration."

Inaudi's memory for figures is stated to have been remarkable. At the end of a performance he was accustomed to repeat all the sums that had been set him. These might amount to 400 figures. He had no power of discovering factors or recognising prime numbers as had Bidder and Colburn.

Inaudi was found by Binet to have an auditory memory. He could remember figures better if he heard them than if he saw them written. But it is a curious fact that, when calculating, he hears the figures in the sound of his own voice. Diamandi, another calculator examined by Binet, had, as is more usual, a visual memory. But what he saw in his mind was not the figures as written but as they would be written in his own handwriting, the 4 and 5 particularly as written by him. When Diamandi takes in a set of figures, two distinct stages were noticed by Binet (1) while he looked at the written figures and (2) while he vivified the image of these figures. No such stages were observable with Inaudi.

Thirdly, it is probable that lightning calculators are aided by their familiarity with the properties of numbers. But such familiarity is not of itself sufficient to produce abnormal calculating power. It is related that on one occasion when the Indian mathematician Ramanujan was lying ill, a friend went to call upon him and happened to mention that the number of his taxicab was 1729, and that he had noticed that this number was equal to $7 \times 13 \times 19$, and he hoped it was not an unfavourable omen. "No," replied Ramanujan, "1729 is a very interesting number : it is the smallest number expressible as the sum of two cubes in two different ways." It has been remarked of Ramanujan that prime numbers seemed to be his personal friends. Despite the familiarity with the properties of numbers thus indicated, no evidence is recorded that he possessed the powers of a lightning calculator.*

An attempt at an explanation of abnormal calculating ability has been made by Scripture. He quotes from De Morgan's *Elements of Arithmetic :* " Learn the multi-

---

* Obituary Notice in *Proc. Royal Society, Series A*, Vol. 99, 1921. The number 1729 is equal to 1^3 plus 12^3 and is also equal to 10^3 plus 9^3.

plication table so well as to name the product the instant the factors are seen, that is, until 8 and 7 or 7 and 8 suggest 56 at once without the necessity of saying 7 times 8 are 56." Thus, in calculating, one may learn to omit " plus," " by," etc., and such shortening of the process, Scripture suggests is the first stage in becoming a lightning calculator. But the omission of such parasite words seems unlikely to carry one far. The mechanical part of mental arithmetic may be quickened, but what the suggestion entirely fails to explain is how a person of low intelligence, like Mondeux, could invent remarkable processes for solving various questions that are ordinarily treated by means of algebra, or how Bidder could instantly recognise the factors of a large number and yet, despite years of study, have failed completely to discover how he attained such a result. We will discuss this point in the following chapter.

Some calculators are slow in their computations. Examples are Buxton and Diamandi. Their capacity was mainly due to an abnormal memory for figures. These cases need not interest us further. Other calculators, such as Bidder and Colburn, produced their results with extraordinary rapidity. This rapidity we have now to investigate. In order to do so it will be necessary for us to make a detour and to consider some instances of other abnormal abilities.

In his book *More Tramps Abroad*, Mark Twain gives a graphic account of a performance, given before the viceroy, by a memory expert who is well-known in India. In one of his feats each member of the audience was asked to think of a sentence, which might be in any language. Then the expert went round the circle and heard from each person the first word of his sentence. Then he made a second circuit and heard each of the second words, and so on. While he was doing this a bell was rung at irregular intervals. When all the sentences had been completed, the expert repeated each sentence complete and also mentioned each occasion on which the bell had been rung.

The explanation given by the expert of this feat was that he imagined a blackboard ruled into spaces. Each word as he heard it he entered in its appropriate space. Recalling the sentences was merely reading out what he saw on his imaginary blackboard. In terms of our simile, this means that, in anticipation of what was coming, the senior clerks had entered the director's room and arranged themselves in a particular order. The incoming impressions were associated because, before their arrival, the senior clerks had become associated. The only association of each impression was its contiguity to the one that had gone before. Such unintelligent association of contiguity is the most harmful and useless kind of memory. A contemporary newspaper report of the performance records a point omitted by Mark Twain, namely, that when the memory expert went away, he forgot his umbrella. In terms of our simile, because the senior clerks were in the director's room, they had no power of sending for other files from the registry. If one of the sentences had been " It is going to rain this afternoon," we may surmise that, even then, no reference would have been made to the registry and that the expert would still have gone away without his umbrella.

The case of the conjuror Houdin has been mentioned, for whom a single glance was sufficient for him to be able to recall a large part of the contents of the window of a toyshop. In this instance we are again dealing with an abnormal readiness of the senior clerks to form associations of contiguity. They differ from the preceding case in that all the impressions were received practically at the same moment. As the senior clerks were already expectant and associated, they had nothing to do but to take in their impressions. There was no possibility of the work of taking in an impression by one clerk interfering with similar work done by another clerk. The impressions arrived practically at the same time. It therefore seems reasonable to suppose that they were taken in by the senior clerks simultaneously.

Thus the speed with which Houdin could remember and recall the contents of a toyshop window was probably due to the fact that different impressions were being recorded simultaneously in different parts of his mind.

Similarly, the speed with which, as we have mentioned, Indian gamblers can count off cowries into fours is explained if we suppose that each group of four was taken in by a different clerk and that the different clerks were carrying on their work at the same time. There is no evidence that they knew the total number of fours. All that was recognised by the gamblers was the number of cowries left over when the rest had been arranged in groups. It has been found by me by experiment that one can separate a number of objects into fours without counting them and find out how many are left over far more quickly than one can count up the total.

A further stage in complication is shown by the ability of Dase to instantly estimate the number of letters in a line of print or the number of a handful of peas thrown on the ground. Here also it is probable that the counting was done in groups and that each group was taken in by a different clerk and that these clerks were all engaged simultaneously.

Bidder suggests that his ability in calculating may have been partly due to his having become familiar with numbers by playing with pebbles or peas before he knew the meaning of symbols. If he heard the number 64, he did not at once think of the symbols 6 and 4. He thought of eight rows of eight pebbles each. In terms of our simile, the junior clerks made an office copy in which the number 64 was represented by eight rows each of eight objects. In this simple case factorising was begun in the act of recognition. It may have happened accordingly that one senior clerk would recognise the factors 8 × 8 while at the same time another saw 16 × 4 and so on. We will return to the question of the importance of factorising in a later paragraph.

The above instances suggest that different acts of recognition and of counting may take place simultaneously in the subconscious mind. We now come to an instance of still more complicated concurrent activities of the subconscious mind.

A case has been related to me in detail of a Madrassi telegraph operator who had the power of listening to four messages simultaneously. He could listen to ticks from four instruments going on at the same time. These ticks were recognised by him as Morse code, translated into letters, sorted into words and then, when the messages were finished, he would call them to consciousness one after the other and write them down. The messages were usually of ten or twelve words each.

Let us now see whether known facts as to the methods used by rapid calculators permit the supposition that their speed was due to different processes occurring simultaneously.

An exceptional instance is recorded in which Colburn found some difficulty in doing a calculation.

It is stated that while in London, on one occasion, " He was asked to tell the square of 4395 ; he at first hesitated, fearful that he would not be able to answer correctly ; but when he applied himself to it, he said it was 19,316,015. On being questioned as to the cause of his hesitation, he replied that he did not like to multiply four figures by four figures, but, said he, " I found out another way : I multiplied 293 by 293 and then multiplied this product twice by the number 15 which produced the same result."

The arithmetic involved in the above explanation is very simple. The numbers 293 and 15 that he used are factors of the number that he had to square.   In other words, 4,395 = 293 × 15.

Colburn, in his memoir, attempts to describe his method of discovering factors.   But, as we shall see, his explanation omits the essential part of the process. and this partial knowledge of his method only became known to his consciousness at a later date.   We may therefore say that Colburn, like Bidder, had an intuitive power of recognising factors.

Consequently we may infer that, while he hesitated, his subconscious mind found that 4,395 was equal to 293 × 15.   But there are other possible pairs of factors for 4,395.   It is difficult to understand how his sub-conscious mind could know which pair was most suitable for use until all these pairs had been discovered and compared.   Therefore it is likely that all the different pairs had been discovered and tested subconsciously. In view of the small amount of time spent on the process, it is probable that in terms of our simile several clerks were at work and that they worked simultaneously. If so, they had the choice of doing the following sums :—

(1)   4,395 × 4,395.
(2)   1,165 × 3 × 1,165 × 3.
(3)   1,165 × 1,165 × 3 × 3.
(4)   1,165 × 1,165 × 9.
(5)   979 × 5 × 979 × 5.
(6)   979 × 979 × 5 × 5.
(7)   293 × 15 × 293 × 15.
(8)   293 × 293 × 15 × 15.

The first four were at once excluded because they

involved multiplying of four figure numbers. Of the others, (8) was found most suitable. Supposing it was worked out by ordinary rules of arithmetic, it would begin with the following multiplication :—

$$
\begin{array}{r}
293 \\
293 \\
\hline
879 \\
2637 \\
586 \\
\hline
85,849
\end{array}
$$

If Colburn had the same kind of visual memory as Mark Twain's expert, then one senior clerk may have been multiplying 293 by 3, while simultaneously another was multiplying 293 by 9 and yet another clerk was multiplying by 2. Before they had finished a fourth clerk may have commenced the next stage, namely, addition of the three lines of figures.

If Colburn had used Inaudi's method he would have multiplied 293 by 293 in stages thus :

$$
\begin{array}{rcrcr}
200 & \times & 200 & = & 40,000 \\
93 & \times & 200 & = & 18,600 \\
200 & \times & 93 & = & 18,600 \\
93 & \times & 90 & = & 8,370 \\
93 & \times & 3 & = & 279 \\
\hline
\multicolumn{5}{r}{\text{Total} = 85,849}
\end{array}
$$

There is no difficulty in supposing that these different multiplications were carried out simultaneously.

The next stage is the addition of the products.   If he used Bidder's method, he would have begun by adding the first to the second, namely, 40,000 to 18,600.   To the product of these two he would have added the third product and so on.   These additions might have begun before the separate multiplications were completed.   The addition of the third to the product of the first two may have been begun before this product was fully obtained. An analogy for such overlapping is to be found among telegraph operators in India who, not infrequently, have the power of beginning to take another message before they have finished writing the address on a message just received.

Colburn's use of factorising is recorded for another sum.   He was asked the product of 21,734 multiplied by 543.   He immediately replied 11,801,562.   But, upon some remark being made on the subject, he said that he had, in his own mind, multiplied 65,202 by 181. Thus he had recognised that 181 is the third of 543 and that it would be an easier figure to use in multiplying.

To summarise the argument.   Reason has been found for suspecting that certain abnormal feats of memory are possible owing to several distinct processes being carried on simultaneously in the subconscious mind. It is possible that when lightning calculators give really instantaneous replies their mental work may have a similar character.   Another and perhaps a more plausible explanation will be suggested in the next chapter.

But the calculations of arithmetical prodigies are not all done instantaneously.   In Gall's account of Colburn we are told that " in calculations at all complicated, he is often heard to multiply, add, or subtract, aloud and with incredible rapidity.

NOTES.

Jedediah Buxton, see *Gentleman's Magazine*, Vol. XXI, 1751, pp. 61 and 347, Vol. XXIII, 1753, p. 557 and Vol. XXIV, 1754, p. 251. He remembered all the free drinks of beer he had had since he was 12 years of age and gave a list of them thus :

D of Kingston	–	–	– 2,130 pints.
D of Norfolk	–	–	266 ,,
Duke of Leeds	–	–	232 ,,
D of Devonshire	–	–	10 ,,
Lady Oxford	–	–	280 ,,
G. Heathcote, Esqr.	–	–	160 ,,
Sir G. Saville Bt.	–	–	20 ,,
&c.,		&c.,	

and so on, amounting to 5,116 pints received from 60 persons.

As regards his method of working :

" He was required to multiply 456 by 378 which he compleated as soon as a person in company had produced the product in the common way ; and upon being requested to work it audibly, that his method might be known, he multiplied 456 first by 5, which produced 2,280, which he again multiplied by 20, and found the product 45,600, which was the multiplicand multiplied by 100 ; this product he multiplied by 3, which produced 136,800, which was the sum of the multiplicand multiplied by 300 ; it remained therefore to multiply it by 78, which he effected, by multiplying 2280 (the product of the multiplicand multiplied by 5) by 15 ; 5 times 15 being 75 ; this product being 43,200, he added to the 136,800, which was the multiplicand multiplied by 300, and this produced 171,000, which was 375 times 456 ; to compleat his operation therefore, he multiplied 456 by 3, which produced 1368, and having added this number to 171,000 he found the product of 456 multiplied by 378 to be 172,368."

Inaudi, see *Psychologie des grands calcalateurs et jouers d'echecs* by Alfred Binet (Paris, Hachette, 1894).

The following example shows his excellent reasoning power in matters of figures :

The question set was, " Find a number of 4 figures whose sum is 25, it being given that the sum of the figures of the hundreds and thousands is equal to the figure for the tens, that the sum of the figures of tens and the thousand is equal to the units figure and if one reverses the number it is increased by 8,082.

Answer : " Since the number increases by 8,082 when reversed, therefore the figure of the thousand must be 1, and the figure for the units 9.   I subtract therefore 9, which is the figure for the units, from 25 ; there remains therefore 16 for the other three figures.   Then the figure for the thousand and that for hundreds are equal to that for tens ; the figure for tens must necessarily be the half of 16, *i.e.*, 8.   Three of the figures being known, it suffices to subtract them from 25 to have that for the hundreds, namely 7, and thus to recognise that the number asked for is 1789."

George Parker Bidder, see his paper " On mental calculation " in *Proc, Institution of Civil Engineers*, London, 1856, Vol. XV, p. 251.   Also Vols. LVII and CIII.

Colburn.   See *The Analectic Magazine*, 1813 (Philadelphia), Vol. I, p. 162, " Remarkable child ; native of America."   This article is reprinted from the *Literary Panorama* (London), Vol. XII, 1813, p. 671.   Also *Memoir of Zerah Colburn written by himself* (Springfield, Merriam, 1833).

The fullest description of abnormal calculating power is that given by Scripture, " Arithmetical prodigies," *American Journal of Psychology*, Vol. IV, April, 1891, p. 1.   Later articles dealing with the subject have usually been written either by persons who have read Scripture's paper and remembered such parts of it as agreed with their preconceived ideas, or are descriptions of isolated cases marred by an undue bias in favour of arriving at an explanation.   Hence it has seemed advisable both to consult and to quote original authorities.

Among queer opinions that have been formed of abnormal calculating power, the following may be mentioned.   Colburn's wonderful gifts convinced " A.B.Esqr., that something had happened contrary to the course of nature and far above it ; he was compelled by this to renounce his infidel foundation, and ever since has been established in the doctrines of Christianity." F. W. H. Myers in *Human Personality* has founded on abnormal calculating power some argument in favour of survival of the soul after death.   Metschnikoff, in discussing human evolution, quoted the instance of Inaudi as an example of a mutation suddenly appearing.   Another queer opinion is to the effect that " It appears to the writer to be probable that any child of IQ (intelligence quotient) over 180 could be taught to be a lightning calculator."

Robert Houdin, *Confidences d'un Prestidigitateur* (Paris, Lbirarie Nouvelle, 1859), Vol. II, p. 9.

CHAPTER V

CALCULATING ABILITY AND INTUITION

Bidder's intuitive power of finding factors—Colburn's discoveries of his methods—Subconscious multiplication—Rhythm—Bidder's methods.

What is an intuition ?   We shall find that an insight into the nature of a particular kind of intuitive power is given us by a further study of calculating ability.

It is recorded by W. Pole that Bidder " had an almost miraculous power of seeing, as it were intuitively, what factors would divide any large given number not a prime.   Thus if he was given the number 17,861, he would instantly remark it was = 337 × 53 ; or he would see as quickly that 1,659 was = 79 × 7 × 3.   He could not, he said, explain how he did this, it seemed like a natural instinct to him."   There can be no doubt that Bidder really had this power.   His son, in a letter to Pole, mentions " My father's great power of seizing instantaneously upon component factors."

Bidder's ignorance of the nature of this power was not owing to his not having thought about it.   In his paper on mental calculation, he tells us that he had studied the subject for years.   The methods of finding factors that he did discover, and that he describes, he regarded as mere matters of curiosity and as of little or no practical use. He makes no pretence of having discovered the method used by his subconscious mind.

Bidder describes the methods used by him in multiplying and in finding square roots. These methods appear to have been practically identical with those used by Colburn. Hence we may infer that the subconscious minds of these two calculators worked in the same way in doing arithmetical problems. Colburn also had an intuitive power of recognising factors. But in his case a partial knowledge of how he did so reached his consciousness some four years after his power had first appeared. Colburn's description, therefore, throws light both on his own and also on Bidder's intuitive power of factorising. His account of his discovery of his method is as follows :

" It was on the night of 9th December, 1813, while in the city of Edinburgh, that he waked up, and, speaking to his father, said : " I can tell you how I find out the factors." His father rose, obtained a light, and beginning to write, took down a brief sketch, from which the rule was described and the following tables formed."

About a year previously, he had become aware of his method of extracting square and cube roots. He says :

" After dinner, Mr. B introduced some mathematical subjects, which he endeavoured to explain to his young understanding. Suddenly Zerah said he thought he could tell how he extracted roots."

Some two years after discovering his method for factors, he became aware of his method of multiplying. This happened, he says, during a visit to Birmingham.

It is singular that the simplest of all his methods should be the last that he was able to explain.

Such detailed description, mentioning time and place, suggests that each discovery, in turn, burst suddenly through into his consciousness. But yet, curiously enough, he says regarding his backwardness in explaining his methods that " it was not owing to ignorance of the methods he pursued ; he rather thinks it was on account of a certain weakness of the mind, which prevented him from taking at once such a general view of the subject, as to reduce his ideas to a regular system in explanation." It is of interest to notice that as soon as he had acquired his general view of the subject, his power of rapid calculation left him finally and completely. It was only so long as his data were not known, or not clearly known, to consciousness that they were fully available for the use of his subconscious mind.

Hitherto Colburn's description of his method of finding factors, which is printed at the end of this chapter, appears to have escaped detailed attention. At first glance it appears to be a dismal juggling with figures to which some unattractive tables are appended. But on looking into it, it appears to be a matter of extraordinary interest.

In the first place, the astonishing fact emerges from his description that, at the age of six years, *before* he had ever discovered a factor or extracted a root, he had done thousands upon thousands of sums in multiplication, and that these sums had not been forgotten but that every detail of them was at the disposal of his subconscious mind. Also it appears that they were classified in a peculiar way. In ordinary multiplication tables the classification is by the numbers multiplied. We put five times one, five times two, five times three, etc., in one table and six times one, six times two, six times three, etc., in another table. In Colburn's subconscious mind the classification was not in this way, namely, by the numbers multiplied : the classification was by the products. For instance he had made the following multiplications :

$$3 \times 67 = 201$$
$$7 \times 43 = 301$$
$$9 \times 89 = 801$$
$$11 \times 91 = 1,001$$
$$13 \times 77 = 1,001$$
$$17 \times 53 = 901$$

His subconscious mind had acted as if it had recognised that each of the above products ended in 01, and had then combined them with other pairs of numbers giving similar products in the following table :

01	01	17	53	31	71	49	49
03	67	19	79	33	97	51	51
07	43	21	81	37	73	57	93
09	89	23	87	39	59	99	99
11	91	27	63	41	61		
13	77	29	69	47	83		

He gives similar tables for every odd number from 01 up to 99, except that he omits numbers ending in 5, as any number ending in 5 is divisible by that number. He omits tables for all even numbers as all even numbers are divisible by 2. Now let us consider how he used such tables in factorising.

Supposing it is required to find the factors of 1401. Because the last two figures of this number are 01, the table above given has to be used. From this table he would arbitrarily chose the pair of numbers 03 and 67. These multiplied together make 201. Then, he says, increase 67 by hundreds, in a series of sums, thus :

$$3 \times 67 = 201$$
$$3 \times 167 = 501$$
$$3 \times 267 = 801$$
$$3 \times 367 = 1,101$$
$$3 \times 467 = 1,401$$

But 1,401 is the number that it is required to factorise. Therefore 3 and 467 are factors of 1,401.

Colburn's understanding of his method is imperfect. Why, it may be asked, did he chose 03 and 67 from the large number of pairs of numbers in the above table ? He gives and he can give no answer. It is tantalising in the highest degree that the information that leaked out from his subconscious mind so narrowly escapes being enough to enable us to understand fully this particular instance of intuition.

The finding of square roots is a particular case of factorising, the condition being that the two factors found should be identical. Hence this method depends on the use of somewhat similar tables. For instance, he had discovered that there are four pairs of numbers, and four pairs only, which being multiplied together yield a product of which the last two figures are 89. These are

$$17 \times 17 = 289$$
$$67 \times 67 = 4,489$$
$$33 \times 33 = 1,089$$
$$83 \times 83 = 6,889$$

His description of his use of these numbers for finding a particular square root is as follows :

" If the square contains six figures, say 321,489, first seek what number squared ends in 89. Answer 67 ; then what number squared comes nearest to 32 ? Answer 5. Combine them—567—which is the root required."

As to why he chose 67 instead of 17 or 33 or 83, he says :

" It is obvious, however, that it requires a good share of quickness and discernment in a large sum, to see which of the four roots . . . is the one to be employed. Such discernment, however, the writer cannot impart."

Thus his knowledge of the method used by his subconscious mind in finding a square root is also tantalisingly defective. His statement that it depends on a good share of quickness and discernment is clearly nothing more than a statement of fact.

For the next step in the explanation we must refer to the records of another calculator—Bidder. There are reasons for believing that he also used tables of " two-figure endings," but little or no knowledge of them seems to have reached his consciousness. He mentions, however, that if called on to extract the square root of 337,561, like Colburn, he would have to choose between four numbers, viz., 19, 31, 69 and 81. He made his choice by recognising similarities. The number 581 was, he says, the square root " inasmuch as 81 stands nearly in the same relation between 500 and 600 as 337,561 does between 250,000 and 360,000, the squares of 500 and 600 respectively.

We have not yet reached the limits of the activity in multiplication of these calculators. Colburn had also carried out multiplications of three identical numbers together. The results were arranged in yet another series of tables which were used in extracting cube roots. As before the classification was by the last two figures of the products.

Why, it may be asked, did Colburn's mind perform the enormous series of multiplications needed to compose his tables ? To say that it was due to " free will " is merely to use a thrionic phrase to conceal our ignorance. Another way of looking at the matter may be suggested.

Multiplication is the process that is the basis of abnormal calculating power. Colburn could multiply, find factors and extract square and cube roots, i.e., do sums involving multiplication, at six years of age, at which time the easier processes of addition and subtraction were difficult to him. The imbecile woman reported by Wizel did addition and subtraction slowly and badly. She was better at division, a process that involves trial multiplications, and she was best at multiplication. She could solve problems in which the number 16 was involved with especial facility, apparently because, in earlier years, she had been fond of arranging and counting objects in groups of sixteen. This effect of repetition of a number suggests that some sort of rhythm was involved.

Multiplication is essentially repetition. Bidder states that he made up for himself a multiplication table long before he knew the use of symbols. For him the fact that eight times eight is sixty-four was not a dogmatic statement learnt from a schoolmaster but it was the result of observation of the product of eight rows each of eight shot or peas. We may imagine that in composing his multiplication table, in this particular instance, one of the junior clerks of our simile got into a kind of rhythmic movement and impressed the image of a row of eight objects eight times on a particular file. Our speculation on this point is in some degree confirmed by the records of another calculator—Mitchell. He tells us that his multiplication was originally counting (*i.e.*, repetition) rather than multiplication proper. When his interest in figures began at three or four years of age, he had no knowledge of multiplication tables. If he wanted to find, for instance, the product of 9×7, he would count 9, 18, 27, etc., up to 63.

Thus the suggestion is made that something in the brain of lightning calculators is apt to indulge in various rhythmic movements and that such movements result in storing records of enormous numbers of sums in multiplication. The vagueness of such a speculation illustrates our ignorance—or, at least, the present writer's ignorance—of the real nature of our mental operations. Arithmetical calculations are among the simplest of our mental processes in that they are are unaffected by sensory impressions arriving at the time or by any other stored data than those relating to figures. Consequently they are well worth the attention of anyone who seeks to discover the physical counterpart of our thought processes.

Bidder gives the following description of his method of multiplying :

" In mental arithmetic you must begin at the left-hand extremity, and you conclude at the unit, allowing one fact only to be impressed on the mind at a time. You modify that fact every instant as the process goes on ; but still the object is to have one fact and one fact only stored away at one time." Clearness of exposition does not appear to have been his strong point. He seems to mean that one fact at a time remains present to consciousness, while other facts are outside consciousness but can be recalled when required. In doing the sum 373×279, he says : " I multiply 200 in 300 = 60,000 ; then multiplying 200 into 70 gives 14,000. I then add them together, and obliterating the previous figures from my mind, carry forward 74,000, etc. . . . the last result in each operation being alone registered by the memory (here he means retained in consciousness), all the previous results being consecutively obliterated until a total product is obtained."

He would use the above method if he was doing a sum consciously. But he could also calculate subconsciously. He says :

" Now, for instance, suppose that I had to multiply 89 by 73, I should say instantly 6,497. If I read the figures written out before me I could not express a result more correctly or more rapidly ; this facility has, however, tended to deceive me, for I fancied that I possessed a multiplication table up to 100 times 100, and, when in full practice, even beyond that ; but I was in error ; the fact is that I go through the entire operation of the computation in that short interval of time which it takes me to announce the result to you. I multiply 80 by 79, 80 by 3, 9 by 70, and 9 by 3 : and then I add them up."

Thus Bidder was in doubt as to the exact nature of the method he employed. Buxton and Inaudi, on the other hand, used slow simple methods that were fully known to their consciousness. Both Colburn and Inaudi were observed to mutter while calculating. Binet overheard Inaudi use such words as " multiplié par " and " je retiens." Such facts suggest that the calculations of Buxton and Inaudi were carried out entirely in consciousness. But yet it is stated that both of them could carry on a conversation while doing their sums. How could they do so if they were consciously attending to their calculations ? Hence it seems probable that their problems were solved sometimes mainly inside consciousness and at other times mainly outside it.

It appears, therefore, that not only is it difficult to know exactly how much of another person's mental processes take place within his consciousness, but, even in the case of a very intelligent man like Bidder, it was difficult for he himself to have a distinct idea of how far his calculations were conscious or subconscious.

A clear proof has also been obtained that thought processes carried out subconsciously may, in some instances, be identical with those carried out in consciousness. In other instances they may differ owing to the fact that stored data may be available to and be used by the subconscious mind that are not available to consciousness. They may differ for another and still more important reason, namely, because the stored data, when in the subconscious mind, are classified differently and have different associations from what they have when in consciousness. In the case of Colburn's calculations, the subconscious classification was the only one of the two that was suitable for use in discovering factors.

That this classification was thus suitable we may regard as a fortunate accident. It was made at the age of six years, at a time when his subconscious mind could have had no inkling that this classification might be used for factorising or for any other purpose. If his multiplications were done consciously, of which we have no definite proof, and had he thought of utility, he, with little doubt, would have put five times one, five times two, etc., in one table and six times one, six times two, etc., in another table. He would have classified his data by the way they were obtained. But when the multiplications passed into his subconscious mind, they were classified by a method that, had he thought about the matter, must have appeared to him as perfectly trivial and useless. Colburn, like other rapid calculators, worked his multiplication sums from left to right. It was the two right hand-most figures alone of each sum, that is to say the figures last obtained, that were used in classifying his results. The classifying must have been a slow process. For instance, when carrying out the multiplications of the numbers 3×1 up to 3×99, he noted that $3 \times 67 = 201$. This was the whole contribution of this particular series of multiplications to his 01 table. Then perhaps some days or weeks later, he would be multiplying 7×1 up to 7×99. While so doing he would note that $7 \times 43 = 301$. This would be his second contribution to his 01 table, and so on.

The conclusion appears to be inevitable that the classification was due to the properties (one is tempted to say physical properties) of his stored data and not to their possible utility in calculating.

Had Colburn, at the time when he was carrying out these thousands of sums of multiplication, thought about the matter, he might have noticed that he was forgetting his results as quickly as he got them. He might have regarded this as regrettable and sought to improve his memory. He could have done this by practice in calling things to mind. Let us consider what would be the result. When we take in a sense impression, at first it is present in consciousness. It then passes from consciousness but can be readily recalled. The impression is now said to be stored in the " preconscious mind." Gradually it passes from the preconscious to the subconscious mind and, when this has happened, it can no longer be readily recalled to consciousness. If every day Colburn had repeated all the calculations he had done the day before, his data would have stayed in his preconscious mind. He would have been able to repeat unintelligently long lists of multiplication sums but he would have acquired this qualification at the cost of his intuitive power. Only when his stored data passed from the preconscious to the subconscious part of his mind would they acquire the classification that was necessary to enable them to be used for rapid factorising. Then they would no longer be available to consciousness for parrot-like repetition of whole tables, but they would not be wholly forgotten for isolated data would still be capable of recall when needed as a step in a reasoned argument.*

Fortunately for Colburn's reputation as a calculator, his data did pass to his subconscious mind at the time. Some years later, still retaining the classification there obtained, they again became available to his consciousness. When this was the case, he could only find factors by employing his tables consciously. As he states in his memoir so doing was "a slow process though a sure one." But, as has been described above, for part of the process, he still had to rely on assistance from his subconscious mind the nature of which he was unable to explain.

* Evidence in favour of this statement may be found in Bidder's description of his discovery of his method of extracting square roots.

The facts brought forward in this chapter permit a suggestion as to the nature of instantaneous common-sense decisions. It is known that impressions forgotten to consciousness are still stored in the subconscious mind and are available to it in the processes of reasoning. Since, in adult life, we have forgotten far more than we can remember, the subconscious mind has at its disposal many more data than has consciousness. This is one reason why, in the more complicated affairs of life, a common-sense intuitive decision is often of more value than one based on conscious reasoning. That it is so rapidly arrived at may be partly due to data stored in the subconscious mind being classified and associated in a far more complicated and comprehensive way than occurs in consciousness.

NOTES.

W. Pole, " Mental Calculation, a reminiscence of Mr. G. P. Bidder, Past President," *Proc. Inst. Civil Engineers, London,* Vol. CIII, 1890-1891, Pt. I, p. 250.

The following is Colburn's description of his method of discovering factors, taken from his *Memoir*, some misprints having been corrected :

" Supposing factors of 1,401 are required ; refer to the table headed 01 ; 01 is of course a common factor to all numbers : take 03 ; as 67 multiplied by 3 gives 201, increase it by prefixing hundreds, and multiplying thus 3 × 167 = 501 ; 3 × 267 = 801 ; 3 × 367 = 1,101 ; 3 × 467 = 1,401. Now if 467 be a prime number, these two are all the factors that will produce 1,401. Consult the table for 67—Will 3 × 89 make 467 ? No. Will 3 × 189 ? No. 7 × 81 exceeds it ; 9 will not divide a number which is not divisible by 3. 11 × 97 exceeds it ; so will 13 × 59. It will be found that 467 is a prime number ; therefore 3 × 467 are the only two factors of 1,401.

Take another number—17,563 ; 03 × 21, with the continual prefix of hundreds and thousands will bring you to 5,821 × 3 = 17,463 ; the addition of another hundred will increase it too much. 07 × 09 = 63 : by the addition of hundreds, etc., you increase 09 to 2,509, which multiplied by 7 gives the proposed sum. Is 2,509 a prime number ? Consult the table for 09 ; after the previous examinations you come to 13, which multiplied by 93, gives 1,209 ; therefore 13 × 7 = 91, which multiplied by 193 will give another pair of factors. Is 193 a prime number ? It will be found such ; therefore 7 × 2,509, and 91 × 193 are the only factors. It may be borne in mind, as an universal rule, that when a simple number will not prove itself a factor, any other number compounded of that simple one will not ; for instance, 21 is formed by 3 × 7 ; if 3 or 7 does not divide the number sought, neither will 21. And also in high numbers, after the right hand figures have been increased by the addition of hundreds and thousands, the left hand figures may be increased in the same manner. It is necessarily a slow process, though a sure one. Again it is not necessary to continue the operation by trying numbers that are above the nearest square root to the sum proposed.''

One of his tables for factorising has already been given, namely, that for 01. He gives similar tables for every odd number up to 99. He says of them that " no notice is taken of the terminations of even numbers ; for they may be divided by two, four, etc., nor yet of 5, as an ending figure of 5 will always divide itself.''

The following are examples of these tables :

Extract from Colburn's tables for finding factors.

09		67		63	
01	09	01	67	01	63
03	03	03	89	03	21
07	87	07	81	07	09
11	19	09	63	11	33
13	93	11	97	13	51
17	77	13	59	17	39
21	29	17	51	19	77
23	83	19	93	23	81
27	67	21	27	27	69
31	39	23	29	29	47
33	73	31	57	31	73
37	57	33	99	37	99
41	49	37	91	41	43
43	63	39	53	49	87
47	47	41	87	53	71
51	59	43	69	57	59
53	53	47	61	61	83
61	69	49	83	67	89
71	79	71	77	79	97
81	89	73	79	91	93
91	99				
97	97				

Extract from Colburn's table for square roots.		*Extract from Colburn's table for cube roots.*	
Square.	Root.	Cube.	Root.
01	01	01	01
	51		
	49	03	47
	99		
		04	34
04	02		84
	52		
	48	07	43
	98		
		08	02
09	03		52
	53		
	47	09	69
	97		
		11	71
16	04		
	54	12	08
	46		58
	96		
		13	17
21	11		
	61	16	06
	39		56
	89		
		17	73
24	18		
	68	19	39
	32		
	82	21	41
25	05	23	47
	15		
	25	24	24
	35		74
	45		
	55	25	05
	65		25
	75		45
	85		65
	95		85
29	27	27	03
	77		
	23	28	12
	73		

Extract from Colburn's table for square roots (cont.).		*Extract from Colburn's table for cube roots (cont.).*	
Square.	Root.	Cube.	Root.
36	06	29	09
	56		
	44	31	11
	94		
		32	18
			68

Colburn's life history as a calculator, briefly and approximately summarised from his autobiography, is as follows :—

Age.

Years.	Months.	
5	11	He could multiply two figure numbers by two figure numbers.
6	2	Multiplying 2 or 3 places of figures, extracting roots and factorising, but weak at addition, subtraction and division.
8	—	Could multiply four places of figures. Was aware of his use of factors in multiplying.
9	—	Occasionally could multiply five or even six places of figures. Discovered the method used by him in extracting roots.
10	3	Discovered method for finding factors.
10	10	Began to learn French.
11	1	Loss of rapidity in calculating, followed by complete loss of his powers.
12	5	Discovered method used in multiplying.

A paper by F. D. Mitchell (" Mathematical Prodigies," *American Journal of Psychology*, January, 1907, Vol. 18, p. 61) is of some interest in that the author is a mathematician who has a limited abnormal calculating ability. He has retained a memory of every stage in the development of his ability. It began with counting. He then went on to counting by 2's and 3's. Then he counted the " power series " of different numbers (2, 4, 8, 16, 32, etc., 3, 9, 27, 81, etc.). But almost always, when the number exceeded 100, he emphasised the last two figures and gradually got into the habit of ignoring the others. Thus instead of saying 3, 9, 27, 81, 243, 729, 2,187, etc., he would count 3, 9, 27, 81, 43, 29, 87, etc. Mitchell gives a full account of Colburn, and doubts Scripture's statement that in adult life he had completely lost his calculating ability. Mitchell says that Colburn's powers were readily revived in 1823 for written longitude computations. But the fact that Colburn could carry out *written* computations is no proof that he had regained his power of rapid *mental* calculation. Colburn in his memoir says of this work that he hoped to improve by practice thus suggesting there was room for improvement. But he appears to have given it up in a very short time.

CHAPTER VI

MUSICAL GENIUS

Precocity of musicians—Uses of music—Musical ability and business ability—Music in education.

In every instance known the power of lightning calculators has appeared at a very early age. Musical genius, in very many if not most instances, is similarly precocious, as shown by the following examples :—*

BALFE, Michael William (1808-1870), composed a polacca at the age of 7.

BEETHOVEN, Ludwig van (1770-1827) went on concert tours at the age of 11.

BELLINI (1802). Father and grandfather were musicians. He began to compose before the age of 6.

BENNETT, Sir William Sterndale (1816-1875), performed a pianoforte concerto of his own at 16.

BISHOP, Sir Henry Rowley (1786-1855), gave early indication of musical talent.

BIZET, Johannes (1833-1897), attracted a good deal of attention as a boy by his compositions and piano playing.

CHERUBINI, Maria Luigi (1760-1842), wrote a successful mass at 13.

* _The Lure of Music_, by Olin Downes (Harper & Brothers, New York and London, 1918), and _The Musical Educator_, Vol. IV, p. 186 (Caxton Publishing Co.).

CHOPIN, Francois Friedrich (1810-1849). " His talent was manifested very early and he had to beware of the hallucinations which music frequently caused him. He began to compose before he knew how to write down his productions."

CLEMENTI, Muzio (1752-1832). In his ninth year accepted a post as organist.

COWEN, Sir Frederick Hymen (1852-   ) composed a waltz at 6 years of age.

CROTCH, Dr. William (1775-1847). The son of a carpenter of musical tastes. At 15 he was appointed organist of Christ Chuich, Oxford.

DEBUSSY (1862). Entered the Conservatoire at 11 and won the Grand Prix at 22.

DIBDIN, Charles (1745-1814). At the age of 15 was engaged as singing actor at Covent Garden Theatre.

FRANCK (1822). " His father exploited him as a youthful prodigy."

GODARD, born 1849, was a child prodigy and afterwards a composer.

GOUNOD (1818). His grandmother was musical. His father was an artist. His mother taught music. At the age of 6 he wrote music to a song.

GRIEG (1843). He writes : " What shall prevent me from calling back that wonderful and mysterious content at discovering, when I stretched up my hands to the piano, not a melody—that was too much—No, but a harmony! First, two notes; then a chord of three notes; then a full chord of four; at last, with both hands—oh! Joy!—a combination of five notes, the chord of the ninth. When I found that my happiness knew no bounds. . . . I was about five years' old." He composed when a schoolboy. But much patient drudgery was needed before he succeeded as a musician.

HANDEL, George Frederick (1685-1759). Played both the organ and the clavier when 7 years old.

HENSCHEL, George (1850). Appeared in public in Berlin as a pianist when twelve years old.

HOFMANN, Josef (1877), became known as a child pianist and afterwards composed.

LEONCAVALLO (1858). His mother was the daughter of an artist. He undertook his first concert tour at the age of 16.

LISZT, Franz (1811-1886). At 9 years of age he already possessed considerable skill as a pianist.

MASCAGNI (1863), " determined, against the wishes of his father, to follow a musical career." At the Conservatory he was a failure having more music in him than concentration or self-control. At 27 he was successful with " Cavalleria Rusticana."

MASSENET (1842). At 11 he went to the Paris Conservatoire. He took the Grand Prix at 21.

MEHUL, Etienne Nicolas (1763-1817). At 11 years of age was organist at his native place.

MENDELSSOHN-Bartholdy, Jakob Ludwig Felix (1809-1847), early showed a great talent for music.

MEYERBEER, Giacomo (1791-1864). Displayed musical talent at a very early age.

MOZART, Maria Anna (1751-1829). " Taken on tour through Europe as a musical prodigy with her brother Wolfgang."

MOZART, Johann Chrysostom Theophilus, commonly called Wolfgang (1756-1791), " excited universal admiration as a child pianist."

NERUDA, Wilhelmina Norman (Lady Halle) (1839). Appeared in public as a violinist at 6 years of age.

OUSELEY, Sir Frederick Arthur Gore (1825-1889). Wrote music when only 8 years old.

PURCELL, Henry (1658). Was one of a family of musicians. He wrote anthems while still a choir boy.

REEVES, John Sims (1818-1900). At fourteen years of age became organist of North Cray Church.

ROSA, Carl August Nicolas (1842-1889). Appeared in public as a violinist when eight years old.

ROSSINI, Gioachino Antonio (1791-1868). At 7 years of age appeared in Paer's opera " Camilla.' At 14 he became musical director of a travelling company.

RUBINSTEIN (1830). At age of 5 his mother noticed how attentively he listened to her piano playing. At 10 he astonished the audience by his performance at a concert.

SAINT-SAENS, Charles Camille (1835). " Commenced to play the piano almost as soon as he could walk."

SCHUBERT, Franz Peter (1797-1828). At 11 played the violin in the school orchestra.

SCHUMANN, Clara Josephine (1819). Made a tour as pianoforte virtuoso at age of 11.

SULLIVAN, Sir Gilbert. " The son of a bandmaster, he learnt to play every wind instrument in the orchestra at the age of eight. His overture to the Tempest was written when he was 18.

THOMAS, Ambroise (1811). " Learned notes with his alphabet."

WEBER, Carl Maria von (1786-1826). His first opera was performed at 14.

ZIMMERMAN, Agnes, Entered Royal Academy of Music at 9.

In appreciating music, in recognising harmonies and in composing, it is probable that processes occur in the brain to which the term rhythmic is applicable. We have suggested that some kind of rhythm may have to do with the development of the abnormal powers of lightning calculators. It is therefore of interest to notice that calculating ability and musical ability resemble each other in their tendency to appear precociously.

A mathematician has told me that mathematicians are always musical. This rule, to which one exception only is known to me, furnishes another indication of the relation between calculating ability and the musical faculty.

Musical precocity may be met with in other clever men besides musical composers. Jeremy Bentham, the utilitarian philosopher, could play the violin at the age of six and retained his taste for music throughout life. It is recorded that he and his brother (who was also a genius) " do not appear to have had a pennyworth of common sense, for common life, between them."

Charles Darwin says that, in Cambridge, he got into a musical set and thereby acquired a strong taste for music. That is to say he enjoyed it. But he had no ear for music ; he could neither recognise a tune nor perceive a discord. In later life, from about the age of thirty, he completely lost his power of enjoying music and also his liking for poetry and his power of enjoying pictures. He says that then, music, instead of giving him pleasure, tended to set him thinking too energetically on whatever he had been working at previously. Aesthetic appreciation probably not infrequently decreases with age. Undergraduates at the University, during their first year, often have a liking for cheap harmony that is a source of trouble to the authorities. In their second and third years the desire for such music, as a rule, greatly diminishes. Similarly, abnormal calculating ability vanishes, as a rule, in adult life. The suggestion is obvious that both musical appreciation and abnormal calculating power are affections of the fallow fields of the mind. William James asserts that " the habit of excessive indulgence in music, for those who are neither performers themselves nor musically gifted enough to take in a purely intellectual way, has probably a relaxing effect upon the character. One becomes filled with emotions which habitually pass without prompting to any deed, and so the inertly sentimental condition is kept up.*

For unmusical people, at all events, one's appreciation of music depends on one's frame of mind. In my own experience, if any difficult matter is occupying my attention, or if it has been occupying my attention on the same day, music is nothing more than a series of disagreeable sounds. The thump, thump, thump of a military march is then more than usually annoying. It appears very differently to the soldiers. Its rhythm accords with the rhythm of their movement and dulls the tedium of marching.

It is easy to find instances of scientific experts, including experts of outstanding ability, who are musical or who enjoy music. But it is less easy to find instances of a similar capacity for enjoyment among successful business men. Indeed, on several occasions, very definite opinions have been expressed to me to the effect that if a man is musical he is no good at business. This may be true of the non-Jewish population in England. But musical ability among prominent Jewish business men appears to be not uncommon. This is of interest

---

* Quoted from *The Psychology of Insanity* by Bernard Hart.

in view of the fact that, in England, Jews appear to be better at arithmetic than the non-Jewish population. The trade in fruit and the trade in precious stones are two occupations that need a large amount of mental arithmetic and both, in London, are almost entirely in the hands of Jews.

What is the use of music, apart from its æsthetic effect ?

One goes to a cinema and finds that the pictures are accompanied by music. If the music stops, the pictures at once seem less pleasing. The explanation commonly given is that the scenes shown, in actual life, would be accompanied by sound. Hence the music remedies the silence of the pictures. This way of looking at the matter will not bear much examination. One still feels the need of the music if the scenes shown are in nature not accompanied by sound, or when they are accompanied by a sound that would drown any imaginable music or when the subject is such that it is impossible to imagine any appropriate music. Let us consider some evidence that will point to a more probable explanation.

Many years ago, Sir William Crookes, the well-known scientist, became interested in spiritualism. He once attended a seance that was conducted by the medium Home. Two other mediums were present, both of whom were afterwards convicted of trickery. The following is an extract from a letter written by him describing this seance :

"Home's singing appeared to drive away the low-class influences and institute his own good ones.

After a minute or two I suggested that we should all sing again, and proposed the song first sung, " For he's a jolly good fellow." Immediately a very sweet voice, high over our heads quite out of the reach of anyone present even had they been standing, and as clear as a bell, said, " You should rather give praise to God." After that we were in no mood for comic songs. We tried something sacred, and as we sung we heard other voices joining in over our heads."

It is astonishing that the author of so many important scientific discoveries, as was Sir William Crookes, did not realise that the music and the frame of mind that it produced was highly unsuited for scientific investigation. The mediums—or at any rate the spooks—knew of one of our mental limitations of which Sir William was unaware, namely that music is not favourable to balanced judgment and that it is frequently used by exploiters of human credulity to dull the reasoning power of their dupes. Music is needed wherever an appeal is made to the emotions rather than to reason.

To return to the cinema ; its pictures are lacking in relief and colour. By the music that accompanies them our judgment is dulled and we become oblivious to their defects and therefore more ready to sympathise with the emotions they evoke. Thanks to the music we can take in the impressions produced by the pictures without criticising them or with less criticism than would otherwise be the case. The music obviously may also act more directly by stimulating the appropriate emotions.

The conductor of a cinema orchestra told me that if, as was often inevitable, the music was not appropriate it was highly necessary that it should be unobtrusive. It failed in its purpose if it distracted the attention of the audience from the pictures.

Thus there can be no doubt that music is unnecessary in an education intended to turn out a business man. There is room for a suspicion that it may be harmful in view of the analogies between abnormal calculating ability and musical genius and in view of the evidence that has been brought forward in a previous chapter that the former ability is usually of the nature of a mental defect.

CHAPTER VII

FORMAL REASONING AND SUBCONSCIOUS JUDGMENT

Normal defects of the human mind—Mechanism for forgetting—
Recollection of school learning—Education and the business
instinct—Mr. X.—Indians and education—Initiative—N—
University Education—Edison—American war Ministers.

Mr. A. E. Morgan, the Principal of the Antioch College, Ohio, has related to me that, on one occasion in a lecture, he illustrated a point by saying that a person driving a motor would probably fail to get through a crowded street crossing if he depended on formal logical processes. Instead of doing this he relies on complicated estimates of the speeds of other cars carried out subconsciously far more rapidly than could be done in consciousness. After the lecture a member of the audience came to him and told him he had in his employ a mathematician who, in his subject, was of exceptional ability. But the bent of his mind was so strong towards formal logical processes that he had had to give up driving his motor. On reaching a crossing he would have to stop and calculate the probability of collisions with other motors. Even his rare mathematical ability was insufficient for such an occasion and he got into so much trouble in driving that he gave up the practice entirely.

This incident illustrates the fact that, if we have to come to a decision, more than one kind of mental process is available.

We may do so by instantaneous intuition. To take the simplest illustration possible, if one has to add up two or three small numbers, one often has, in my experience, an immediate intuition of what the total will be. Scripture taught himself to recognise instantly the total of two numbers before he had consciously grasped the value of either.

Or we may come to a decision by a process of consciously weighing the evidence. This process is better called " formal reasoning " than " conscious reasoning." because it is probably aided in different ways, and to different degrees in different cases, by activities of the subconscious mind.

With more complicated affairs, neither the immediate intuition nor immediate conscious reasoning may suffice to lead us to a definite conclusion. One follows the popular advice to sleep over a matter before deciding. On waking in the morning, a fresh opinion may come at once, or with little effort into consciousness. Even then we cannot be sure that we have arrived at our final belief. If we return to the subject six months later, we may find that reasons which previously seemed conclusive now seem to us of negligible importance and again we may arrive at another opinion.

This last fact reminds us both of the imperfections of our thinking mechanism and of the defects of our attempted description of the reasoning process. The simile used in a previous chapter took no account of the prejudices, the feelings, the complexes and the results of past experience that constantly influence our decisions and our conduct.

Helmholz once asserted that the eye, regarded as an optical instrument, has almost every possible defect. This is of little moment to us in practical affairs, as we see not with the eye but with the brain, and the brain, without our knowing it, compensates for the defects of its instrument. But we have no higher monitor to compensate for the defects of our thinking mechanism, to warn us when a preconceived idea makes us reject valid reasoning or when some longed-for object leads us to accept imperfect reasoning as conclusive.

The mind has yet another defect. For some purposes formal reasoning is the better and for other purposes intuition. But we have little or no power of deciding which we shall use. A cricketer tells me that when batting to a slow bowler, he decides consciously how to hit the ball. When batting to a fast ball, he decides subconsciously and his subconscious judgment, he asserts, is the better of the two. But he has no choice in the matter. If there is time he must use reason. Only if time is insufficient for formal reason does the " spur of the moment " stimulate his subconscious mind to come to his aid.

An example of the rare occasions when some sort of choice is possible between conscious and subconscious mental activity is in my own experience of using a typewriter. If, by a conscious effort, I do not look at the keys, it is possible for me to type without doing so. But to do so successfully, it is necessary for me to write quickly and without thinking about what I am doing. Hesitation or trying to think of the position of the keys at once leads to mistakes. Thus a set of impressions, namely, knowledge of the position of the keys, may be known to me consciously or subconsciously. It is only when this knowledge is excluded from consciousness by a mental effort that it is fully available for use by the subconscious mind.* Similarly Bidder asserted that confidence was necessary for success in his mental calculations. That is to say, his subconscious mind could be spurred into activity by suggestion.

My readers probably can recall occasions when they were unable to decide beforehand what to say in an interview, but yet when, at the moment of the interview, the right words came suddenly to consciousness. Similarly " Necessity is the mother of invention."

In the case of the cricketer above mentioned, the power of deciding consciously put his subconscious mind out of action (that is, so far as known decisions were concerned). This is an example of what seems to be a general rule. Those whose capacity for formal reasoning is abnormally developed are apt to use such reasoning on occasions when common sense would be more suitable. Not only can we not expect to develop common sense by

---

* Some savages have a remarkable power of rapid decision in mechanical matters, as for instance when guiding a canoe in rapids, but lack the power of rapid decision in social or intellectual affairs. Such a fact suggests the possibility that the abnormal size of the human brain is partly due to its having been evolved originally for aiming or throwing stones or other weapons and that it had only secondarily been adapted for the higher powers of thought.

practice in formal reasoning but we may anticipate that any such practice, if carried too far, would tend to check the development of common sense.

It is known to psychologists that the power of forgetting is an important part of our mental equipment. Facts recorded in the preceding chapter and other facts to be mentioned later indicate that so long as the data are within easy reach of consciousness they are inevitably used in conscious reasoning. Data only become available to the subconscious mind when they have been forgotten or are so vaguely remembered (as occurs with a jury) that they are no longer capable of being used in a consciously reasoned argument. Hence it appears that the act of forgetting is a necessary condition for subconscious judgment. Hence also it is probable that artificial stimulation of memory by the schoolmaster, so far as this harms the mechanism for forgetting, must tend to add to the power of conscious reasoning only at the expense of our power of subconscious judgment. More than three hundred years ago Montaigne said in his essays that it is commonly seen by experience that good memories do rather accompany weak judgments. We will now adduce other facts that appear to offer an explanation of Montaigne's observation.

Although activity of the subconscious mind may play a part in every act of so-called conscious reasoning, this must not blind us to the fact that in practice there is a wide difference between the mental habit of the expert, who perforce must use conscious reasoning in his work and that of the man of business who has similarly to depend on common-sense decisions in which conscious reasoning plays but little part. Not only are there differences but also, as will be shown in later chapters, a certain amount of incompatibility between these two modes of thought.

Evidence is available that the expert generally remembers for a longer time things learnt with effort than does the practical man. For instance, every expert questioned by me on this point, when in middle life, was found to be able to recall a good deal of what he had learnt at school. An expert, who sometimes forgot whether or not he had had his breakfast, was able to recall much Latin and Greek, though he had had no occasion to call these subjects to mind since he was a boy. He could, he assured me, repeat by heart whole pages of Latin authors. On one occasion a geological expert was talking to me on some geological matter. Presently he got out of his depth and excused himself by saying he had got rather rusty on geological matters, having been away for the last two years, first at the war in Mesopotamia and afterwards on munition work. On my then asking him what he remembered of his school learning, he was able to recall some Latin, Greek and Euclid just as well as other experts.

On the other hand, men of business generally, when in middle life, have completely forgotten their school learning. One has been quoted who had taken prizes for mathematics but who was unable to define parallel straight lines. Others were unable to recall a single word of Latin or the title of a single proposition of

Euclid. An engineer was similarly unable to recall any Euclid, which, as he said, was remarkable, since he was constantly using geometrical methods in his work. An interesting exception to this rule was a business man who seemed to be unusually intelligent. He has been heard by me to make a Latin quotation that was not at all hackneyed and also to criticise someone else's quotation in a way that showed that he retained a working knowledge of the Latin grammar. He was full of ingenious schemes for making money. But they never succeeded. His reasoning power was good but he completely lacked the business instinct and his name was said to be synonymous with failure.

A few instances have come to my knowledge of business men and members of the Indian Civil Service who keep up an interest in the classics. One civilian told me that though he enjoyed reading classical authors he had completely forgotten all details of grammar and syntax. More frequently Indian civilians have forgotten their classics and have great difficulty in recalling even the names of the subjects they took up for their entrance examination.

Cases of memory of school learning in after life occur among administrators and statesman of unusual ability. As an example we may refer to William Pitt who became Prime Minister of Great Britain at the early age of twenty-six. He was distinguished for his eloquence. When asked how he had acquired the power of finding the right word, when speaking, always without pause or hesitation, he replied that he believed that such power as he had in this respect was greatly owing to a practice that he had learnt from his father (Lord Chatham). It was to take up a book in some foreign language with which he was acquainted, in Latin or Greek especially. Lord Chatham enjoined him to read out a passage translating into English, stopping, where he was not sure of a suitable word, until the right word came to him, and then to proceed. Mr. Pitt said that he had followed this practice assiduously. If we admit that the eloquence of Mr. Pitt and Lord Chatham was due to this exercise, the matter is of some interest, for it is commonly believed that calling things to mind only improves the memory indirectly, namely, by causing a habit of increased attention when taking in impressions. But the practice in question, if it was of use, must have been so by giving increased facility in calling to mind impressions that had been taken in, perhaps years previously, before the exercise had begun, and when, therefore, there was no possibility of any artificially increased attention. In this case we are not dealing with the recall of a single impression, as would be the case if one tried to remember whether one had had an egg for breakfast. The case is the more striking because we are dealing with recall of one chosen from a number of stored impressions. This choice probably could not have been good until practice had given to the subconscious mind an increased power of choosing between its stored impressions.

Abundant proofs that experts generally lack the business instinct will be found in later chapters. It will be shown that in almost every instance in which an expert has shown business capacity he has been a business man first and has acquired expert aptitudes later. The highly developed reasoning power of the expert involves a habit of remembering the facts about which he has to reason. If what one forgets subserves the subconscious mind one would anticipate that this habit of remembering would be hostile to the appearance of the business instinct.

If forgetting is a necessary prelude to the activity of the subconscious mind (*i.e.*, for subconscious judgment), then, since the main apparent object of education is to develop memory, one would expect it to be possible to show that a good education is hostile to the development of the business instinct. Evidence to this effect is readily available.

Let us first consider an example of a mode of arguing that should be avoided.

In a debate on an Education Bill in the British Parliament in 1918, a member expressed himself as follows : " It was said that education was necessary to make the rising generation good business men. His experience in the city was that the man who took firsts at Oxford generally came out last and the man who could hardly write his name generally came out first. The explanation was that education could not put into a man that instinct of self-preservation and common sense which was the foundation of success in business. How could education assist a farm labourer

to spread manure on a field ? The best labourer he
had known was wholly illiterate. If the waste of war
was to be replaced it would be necessary for the young
to start as early as possible in doing a day's work,
instead of wasting time on useless book learning."

This pronouncement reminds one of Lord Mansfield's
advice never to give reasons. The judgment of this
Member of Parliament, as we shall see, is probably
right, but his reasons are certainly wrong. The case of
the farm labourer is no good reason for not giving a
good education to a business man.

His judgment was quoted by a very distinguished
scientist as an illustration of " the stultifying effect of
a purely classical education," the Member of Parliament
in question having been educated at " one of the most
rigidly classical of our public schools."* It will be of
interest to see in what this stultifying effect consists.
The speaker can scarcely have meant that there had
been any stultifying effect on such subconscious mental
powers as common sense, business acumen, or initiative,
for he describes the Member of Parliament in question
as being a director of one of the largest London banks
and of one of the most important English railways.
The stultifying effect, if not on the instinctive intuitive
powers of the mind, must have been on its more
conscious activities, namely on its power of formal
reasoning. Certainly, in the example quoted, the reasoning of this Member of Parliament is of a kind more

* *Journal of the Chemical Society*, April, 1918, p. 894.

suited for debate than for scientific discussion. He gives an explanation that can be easily criticised ; he assumes that no answer is possible to a question that he propounds ; he makes a somewhat rash and sweeping statement about " useless book learning." How does he know that the limited classical education he received was not of use, in that, by checking the precocious development of conscious reasoning, or in some other way, it may have stimulated the capacity for subconscious mental activity ? The power of formal logical reasoning and the power of subconscious judgment vary inversely to such an extent that it is by no means an irrational enquiry whether the discipline of dull and useless book learning that is bad for one is not good for the other.

But the scientific critic of this Member of Parliament may himself be criticised. He gives an example of a man of classical education who was manager of a large bank and an important railway. He thinks that scientific is better than classical education. Then why does he not quote an instance of a manager of a still larger bank and a still longer railway who had been scientifically educated ? On another occasion the same distinguished scientist criticised publicly a certain notorious quack medicine. One of his arguments against it was that no instances could be brought forward of the use of this medicine having resulted in a cure. What is sauce for the goose is sauce for the gander. If such proof is demanded in the case of a quack medicine, why is it not given in the case of scientific education ? Perhaps no such proofs were present to his consciousness. The reason why this was probably the case is a matter that we have now to investigate.

Let us begin by considering instances in which proof is available that education is of use in business or commercial affairs.

Evidence may readily be found of the advantage to a business man of a good education in those businesses in which rapid initiative and business instinct are not required from beginners. For instance, educational qualifications are especially relied on in admitting candidates into the banking business and an experienced banker has informed me that he has noticed that boys who have done well at school do better as bankers than boys whose school life was not so promising. When boys first enter a bank, obedience and accuracy are far more useful to them than initiative and enterprise. At first beginners are put to do routine work of the simplest kind. One, it may be, for some years, has no other duty than to add up columns of figures ; another is occupied in writing up pass books ; another has to take charge of addressing and despatching letters. If a beginner shows aptness in his work, the head of his department will make a point of changing him at intervals from one kind of work to another. But whatever he does it is all dull routine. After some years of dull discipline of this kind, without any further preparation, the young banker is suddenly promoted to the position of manager of a branch of the bank. Thus after a training in which he has no opportunity of exercising his initiative, he is put in a position in which he is expected to show, and generally does show, this power of the mind. Thus he exhibits the power of deciding in business matters, not after practice in deciding, but after what may be described as practice in forgetting, for his dull work in adding up figures, precisely because it makes so little appeal either to his interest or to his conscious reason, is of a kind that is instantly forgotten.

On the other hand it is probable that in banking, as in other affairs, routine work of one kind, if too long continued, is bad for the mental powers. Certain evidence, of a kind not convenient to quote in detail, has led me to the suspicion that this is especially the case in occupations the preparation for which involves much stimulation of intelligence and memory.

Large engineering firms, in some cases, only admit men with university degrees in technical subjects. Such men do well in the positions in which they find themselves, but their work at first is mainly technical and they are not required to do work for which business instinct is required. An engineer of wide experience told me that he once had under him a man with a university degree. This man was admirable, he said, for designing a suspension bridge or any work of that kind but " he was no earthly use at commercial engineering."

We will now consider evidence that ordinary school education is hostile to the development of the business instinct.

Stephen Leacock thus sums up his experiences as a schoolmaster in Canada : " I have noted that of my pupils those who seemed the laziest and the least

enamoured of books are now rising to eminence at the
bar, in business, and in public life ; the really promising
boys who took all the prizes are now able with difficulty
to earn the wages of a clerk in a summer hotel or a deck
hand in a steamboat."*

At a meeting of the Association of Technical Institutions held in July, 1924, Alderman J. Q. Guy, chairman
of the Bradford Education Committee, stated that in
some way secondary school training absolutely unfitted
a boy for picking up the special sense required for wool
buying. Mr. W. M. Rankin, principal of Burnley
Municipal College, in the course of a discussion, said
that there seemed to be something in the atmosphere
of higher education that inhibited the industrial capacity
of members of families engaged in commercial activities.
He referred to the common belief in industrial centres
in the north of England that the quickest way to end a
firm is to send their boys to a public school or university
A report to this effect was published in the *Daily Mail*.
A few days later it published interviews with two large
employers of labour to the effect that they found
advantage in employing university men in their business.
There can be little room for doubt that this must be the
case as regards employees in subordinate positions.
They will be more intelligent, more accurate, more
industrious perhaps, more dependable and more pliable
than men who have not had such an education. Perhaps
there will be an additional advantage. They will not

---

* Preface to *Sunshine Sketches of a little Town.*

be likely to run away and found a rival business. They will lack the initiative. Perhaps they are also likely to lack the business instinct that would qualify them to become the head of the firm that employs them.

It has already been stated that certain large firms of engineers only admit employees, of course for their higher branches, who have university degrees in technical subjects. Similarly this is no proof that such employees have the business instinct that would be required to enable them to take the position of head of the firm. Mr. Herbert Spencer says : " It is astonishing how general, among distinguished engineers, has been the absence of education, or of high education. James Brindley and George Stephenson were without any early instruction at all : the one taught himself writing when an apprentice, and the other put himself to school when a grown man. Telford, too, a shepherd boy, had no culture beyond that which a parish school afforded. Though Smeaton and Rennie and Watt had the discipline of grammar schools, and two of them of high schools, yet in no case did they pass through a curriculum appropriate to the profession they followed. Another piece of evidence, no less remarkable, is furnished by the case of Sir Benjamin Baker, who designed and executed the Forth Bridge : the greatest and most remarkable bridge in the world, I believe. He received no regular engineering education."*

It may be noted that none of these were men who

---

* Herbert Spencer's *Autobiography*, Vol. I, pp. 167 and 337.

joined large firms in which they slowly worked their way up. They were men who struck out their own line, with whom, therefore, there was demand for initiative and ambition from the start, with one exception. The exception was James Watt who was an inventor rather than an engineer. He said of himself: " I am not enterprising. I would rather face a loaded cannon than settle an account or make a bargain." Fortunately he got into partnership with a business man—Boulton— who wisely left invention to Watt while he himself took charge of the actual business. Watt was distinguished for his fund of general knowledge. Thus unusual power of formal reasoning (shown by his inventive capacity) and unusual memory (shown by his general knowledge) was combined with great lack of initiative.

Sir Joseph Isherwood, whose method of longitudinal construction has inaugurated a new era in shipbuilding, left school at the age of fifteen and " plunged at once into hard work as a ship's draughtsman."

Sir Alfred Yarrow left school at $15\frac{1}{2}$, obtained a post as a mechanic, gradually worked his way up and at length originated works for buiding torpedo boats of world-wide reputation.

The education of G. P. Bidder was much interrupted, as his father, who was a stone-mason, used to take him about the country to exhibit his remarkable powers of mental calculation. In spite of this supposed handicap, he became a distinguished engineer and was the builder of the East India Docks in London.

Mr. A. E. Morgan of Antioch College informs me that there is a saying among American engineers that an engineer tends to fail as a contractor. The engineer is well educated and possesses the scientific knowledge necessary for his work. The contractor is comparatively badly educated and has common sense and business capacity. Mr. Morgan says that " the contractor, on the other hand, who has started out in life as water boy, become a labourer and then a foreman and finally gone to work for himself, in all of his experiences has had many exigencies to meet. He has not been prepared to meet them by formal analysis (owing to his bad education) and many of them did not lend themselves to that type of solution. He has therefore developed this second sense of intuition or judgment as a guide. In the practical carrying out of his work, he finds many more occasions where this intuition is a sure guide than he does where analysis is a sure guide. Hence for the contractor intuition is of more value than the power of formal analysis."

It is quite a usual statement in the biographies of self-made men that they resolved that their sons should have a good education, they themselves having been, as they assert, greatly handicapped by the lack of it. If, as usually seems to happen, the sons fail to distinguish themselves in business, this is not a sufficient proof that their education has checked the growth of their business instinct, for it is possible that they have been handicapped by their lacking the stimulus to exertion that had aided their fathers. On the other hand the conditions are different if we have to deal with two brothers who are under an equal necessity of pushing their way and who differ in their educational advantages. If one is well educated and shows no business instinct and the other is badly educated and shows this power, then we have evidence to the point. Four such instances have come to my notice, two of which are worth describing in detail.

In an earlier chapter a business man of my acquaintance was quoted as Mr. X. The following is a further account of his mental equipment.

Mr. X had a bad school education because it was constantly interrupted by long periods of ill health. It was only at the age of eighteen that he found himself with a good constitution.

He was then apprenticed to a manufacturer and showed sharpness, energy and initiative. He was selected to represent the firm as a travelling agent, and, at present, is a foreign " commission agent " for several firms dealing with various kinds of manufactured articles.

As his memory has never been developed to any great degree by his school education, he has no aptitude for languages. As a young man he felt the handicap of having a bad memory so he determined to improve it. This he did by writing out at night all he could remember of the accounts and orders he had had to do with during the day. He was so successful at this that he can now remember orders or promises that he made two years previously.

But this memory is entirely special and limited to this one thing. He frequently forgets whether he has had his lunch.

An unusual characteristic in a business man is that Mr. X is a great reader of books, and, when travelling, he carries his library catalogue with him. This he showed me. It appeared to be remarkably well chosen. It contained books relating chiefly to sociology, history, history of religion, travel and the geography of the countries he was in the habit of visiting.

Mr. X has the power of forgetting in a remarkable degree, so much so that if he sees the title of any of his books he is unable to recall the contents. Like other business men he has forgotten all he learnt at school. He was unable to quote a single Latin word when challenged to do so. But yet, though he has forgotten the French and Latin he learnt as a boy, what he learnt, he says, helps him in understanding a few French or Italian phrases when travelling in countries where these languages are spoken. What he remembers depends very much on the environment. He knows a few words of Hindustani but can only recall them when in Northern India. He could not, he said, recall a single word of Hindustani when travelling in Madras where that language is not spoken. He asserted that though he forgot the contents of the books he read, some of what he had learnt would come back to him when he wanted it. On my then asking him whether the Malayan fire-piston (a primitive method of producing fire) was mentioned in any of his books, he told me with confidence that it was not referred to in Fraser's *Golden Bough* or in books by Wallace or by Skeats and Blagden. Though he showed some memory in this case, as a rule, the stimulus of conversation was not sufficient to recall to his consciousness anything more than the vaguest conceptions of the contents of the books he had read. His conversation consisted of the usual mixture of trivialities with a few shrewd remarks that one would expect from a business man. Mr. X is not a plausible or excessive talker. He appears to hold a prominent position in his line of business. Another business man gave me independent evidence of his ability.

His interests are limited to matters that affect his pocket. A recognised stimulus to memory is interest. One is more likely to remember what is interesting than what is uninteresting. Mr. X, in spite of his capacity for forgetting things that are unimportant to him, has a good memory for things in which he is interested such as the details of his business. He once was offered an agency in certain hardware manufacturers. He accepted on the condition that he should be allowed to spend four days at the factory learning technical details. This he did and learnt up the subject thoroughly. He gave me a somewhat detailed account of an instance in which this technical knowledge had been of great use to him in India.

Thus Mr. X presents an instance of great business ability, initiative and power to learn new things or take up new lines of work in a man who had had a bad school education. The following description of a brother of

Mr. X, whose school education had been good, will serve as a sort of control observation.

This man had a well-developed memory. He acquired an expert turn of mind and became an analytical chemist. He obtained a post with a company that sold a certain product made in plantations in various eastern countries. As his memory was well trained, he had no difficulty in learning well six languages spoken by various people he met while in the east. Also in virtue of his good memory he was able to become expert in estimating the value of the shares of various companies dealing in the product in which he was interested. Owing to his knowledge he made a good deal of money by speculating in these shares and has given up his chemical work. He has been able to do this, not owing to any business instinct, but as a result of sheer hard work, memory, and logical reason. Owing to his lack of the business instinct, though he knows what to buy, he sometimes does not know when to sell. Conscious reason may show that certain shares are likely to rise, but, as Mr. X informed me, conscious reason would be insufficient, and business instinct would be needed to determine when the rise was coming to an end and when it was about to be followed by a fall. He has made a fortune, lost it and made another. He is not adaptable. He has little initiative and is only good at this one thing, namely, knowledge of a certain class of shares on which he is a recognised authority.

Thus, of these two brothers, one had a good education, a good memory and no business instinct ; the other had a bad education, a bad memory, though a useful one, and a highly developed business instinct.

A similar example is to be found in the life of George Moore, merchant and philanthropist. George Moore was a country boy of bad education who came to London and pushed his way. He was acutely conscious of the handicap of his bad education and wrote to his father urging him to give his younger brother William the best education obtainable. " It is," he wrote, " the best thing you could furnish him with in setting out in the world. It is better than money. Education will enable him to start fair in the world and to push his own way. His biographer says : " William was accordingly sent to the best schools. He was a far apter learner than George had been. He had read extensively, and was well versed in literature. But he wanted that in which his brother George was supreme, intense perseverance. He knew much and did little. He could think but could not work. Nevertheless, George had much confidence in his brother William, because of his superior education and his extensive knowledge." If this statement is true the confidence appears to have been somewhat misplaced ; for William had neither perseverance, nor business instinct, nor initiative, the qualities for which his badly educated brother was specially distinguished.

Indians have an unusual capacity for developing the memory by practice. It is only in India that one hears of a money lender who, being illiterate, keeps all his accounts in his head, or of an accountant to a bank who depends on memory except for a few marks on a wall made with a piece of charcoal.   Such abnormal memory appears to be entirely special to one class of data.   The Indian student, who arouses the despair of his schoolmaster by learning a textbook by heart, without having properly assimilated its contents, is by no means distinguished for general knowledge.   A distinguished Indian judge once told me the following story : A student in an examination was asked a question that he did not properly understand but he felt sure that the answer was included in one or other of two paragraphs of his textbook.   He accordingly wrote them both out *verbatim*—no difficult task as he knew the book by heart. He was ploughed and it was only some years afterwards that he had sufficiently recovered from the effects of his education for him to be able to understand that his examiner was in the right.

The proofs that we find in India of the bad effects of undue stimulation of memory are the more valuable in that the intellectual ability of the mature Indian mind is undoubted.   The opinion is widely held that western education has not yet done full justice to the Indian mind.

The celebrated Bengali chemist, Sir Prafulla Ráy, after quoting the phrase that " our university made a havoc of originality," stated that most of the prominent men in Bengal have no university degrees.   The late Dr. Annandale, in giving evidence before the Calcutta University Commission, said : " I have never in my own department appointed as a clerk or assistant any man who had a university degree. . . . It has been my experience that I could engage better men by ignoring university qualifications. . . . By better men I mean, not men who were better acquainted with rules and regulations or more capable of assimiliating official routine, but men who were better able to adapt themselves to changing conditions and different kinds of work, even if their actual powers of intellect were not so highly trained."*

Among the different races in India the business instinct is rarely, if ever, met with in members of the more intellectual and better educated classes. On the other hand Mahomedans and Marwaris, who have had a very bad education, often are extremely capable in business. All the wholesale trade in certain articles in Calcutta and Bombay is in the hands of Mahomedan merchants.

Sir Prafulla Rây, in a speech on the industrial position of India, referred to " the illiterate persons of East Bengal who made handsome incomes from jute and other businesses and to the Marwaris and Bhattiahs who had almost ousted the Bengalees from the Calcutta industrial market. . . . The Bengalees would not count for more than four per cent. in the business market of Calcutta."†

Mr. L. K. Ananta Krishna, Superintendent of the Ethnographical Survey of Cochin State in southern

---

* *Calcutta University Commission Report*, 1917-1919, Vol. X, p. 112.

† Reported in the *Times of India*, weekly edition, April 30th, 1919.

India, tells me that the Mahomedans in Cochin are known as "Moplahs." They originated from the union of Arab immigrants with women of the soil. Their mother tongue is Malayalam. Their education is next to nothing. They can read Arabic, but there are no scholars among them. They know enough arithmetic to calculate interest. They are good business men. The trade in hides is mostly in their hands. They predominate in both wholesale and retail trade in paddy, coir, copra, European manufactured commodities, pepper, timber, and other local products. Mr. Ananta Krishna says that, in southern India, educated Hindus may be found in retail but never in wholesale trade.

In other parts of India the business instinct is specially shown by members of the Baniya caste whose education consists almost entirely of commercial mental arithmetic. The disastrous effects on their business ability of replacing such education by a rational education will be described in a later chapter.

It is a curious fact that a large number of prominent American men of business began their careers as telegraph operators. This statement is made in a book called *Edison, His Life and Inventions*. Sending messages with a Morse key is not, as yet, a recognised means of developing the business instinct, nevertheless a list is given in this book of twenty-one celebrated men of business, railways directors, etc., besides Edison himself, each of whom began his career in this way. There can be little doubt that each of these men had nothing more than a restricted school education, but yet they were able to compete in business against others often more learned than themselves. Sending and receiving telegrams is work that involves taking in impressions rapidly that are as rapidly forgotten. Hence practice in forgetting, in an usual amount, was, in these cases, followed by an unusual development of qualities that lead to success in business such as initiative and the business instinct.

Anyone who has had much practice in forgetting, if he has to deal with a difficult subject, is likely to take it in with exertion but yet, despite his exertion, to be able to forget it rapidly. As we have seen it is the forgotten impressions (*i.e.*, forgotten to consciousness) that are at the disposal of the subconscious mind and are used by it in acts of subconscious judgment. If this conclusion is correct, one would expect evidence to be available that too good a memory is detrimental in those occupations in which subconscious judgment rather than formal reasoning is required. In order to put this matter to a test, the following question was submitted to a large number of men : " Do you know of anyone with exceptional memory and reasoning power who, in spite of these qualities, is not successful in his work ? Everyone asked this question has been aware of instances to the point and everyone without exception has put his finger on the same mental defect. The following are the last six consecutive replies received by me at the time of beginning to write this chapter :

(1) An officer, who had had a great deal to do with training officers for the new army in the great war, told

me that the most unsatisfactory material for making officers out of, was schoolmasters. They were men of intelligence, ahead of others in book-learning and in capacity to learn. But when turned into officers they were useless because they completely lacked initiative. On later occasions, two other officers have given me identical opinions. This evidence goes to show that officer schoolmasters are at fault in positions in which rapid decisions were required. An account of another officer schoolmaster has been given me who held an appointment in which he had to draw up elaborate schemes for submission to his superiors. Such work demanded reasoning, foresight and originality rather than sudden decisions and these qualities he showed in a remarkable degree.

(2) The manager of the largest bank in one of the British Dominions told me he knew a man who was extremely expert in the theory of banking and in various problems of economics. He enjoyed visiting this man to have a chat with him on such subjects. But in actual business this man was " an absolute fool. He had no initiative."

(3) An engineer told me of an engineer of his acquaintance who was exceptionally full of book-learning. If methods of making such a thing as a culvert were discussed, he would describe the method adopted by English engineers and show how it differed from the methods employed by American, French or Italian engineers. One day he was sent to make a culvert. It was at the side of a hill. He commenced by taking

down a retaining wall that supported the side of the hill and was in his way. Presently it began to rain. The hill started subsiding and the only thing to do was to put back the retaining wall as quickly as possible. But this did not occur to him. Nothing occurred to him. He telegraphed for assistance. On this as on other occasions he showed that he completely lacked what my friend called the "engineering instinct." Here again was an instance of too much learning accompanied by lack of initiative.

(4) The fourth person asked said he knew of many instances of men having much reasoning power and no initiative. He did not quote any particular case. He was an administrative officer of great common sense and a memory quite unburdened with useless information.

(5) An acquaintance who had been to a certain school told me it was notorious that the education there was so good that its boys were constantly getting scholarships and exhibitions at the universities. But it was also notorious that one never seemed to hear of these boys afterwards. He told me of one case of an exceptionally "clever" man, who had been at this school, who passed first into some government department, but who "hadn't got sufficient initiative to tie up his bootlace. If you asked him to go for a walk, he would reason about it for ten minutes before he could decide what to do."

(6) The last was an official and gave the same sort of reply as (4).

In view of the many opinions collected by me, it

appears that the fact that people with too much memory and reasoning power are deficient in initiative may be described as something that everyone knows and that nobody realises.

Edison is recorded as saying, " What we need are men capable of doing work. I wouldn't give a penny for the ordinary college graduate, except those from the institutes of technology. Those coming up from the ranks are a darned sight better." To a question as to where he found the best young men to train as his assistants, in an interview with Mr. Poulteney Bigelow, he answered emphatically : " The college-bred ones are not worth a d——. I don't know why, but they don't seem able to begin at the beginning and give their whole heart to the work." In commenting on this opinion, Mr. Herbert Spencer says that the evidence available leads to the inference that the established systems of education, "whatever their matter may be, are fundamentally vicious in their manner."

America seems to have followed Edison's advice in choosing men " capable of doing work " for the heads of various organisations needed in connection with the war. We may well believe she picked her best men. Of these, Mr. Danield Willard, who was in control of all transportation work, began life as a railroad labourer, then worked as an engine driver and gradually rose to his present position. Mr. Vanderlip, a banker, was the chairman of the British War Loan Committee in the United States. He then became assistant to the Treasury Secretary. He is the chief of the sixth biggest

bank in the world. He began life as a reporter. Mr.
Rosenwald, who was in charge of "war buying of
finished products," began life as an errand boy. He
belongs to a large mail order house in Chicago and is
reputed to have an income of a million dollars a year.
Mr. H. P. Davison, a banker, formed a committee of
of bankers to help in war organisation. As he made
£200,000 before he was twenty years of age, he could
not have spent any undue time on his education. Mr.
John D. Ryan, Director of Aircraft Production, is said
to be a self-made man. He is pre-eminent in industrial
organising power. Mr. Robert Lovell, "a kind of
reconstruction minister" also rose from the ranks. Mr.
Charles M. Schwab, Director-General of the United
States Emergency Fleet Corporation, as a boy drove
a stage hackney carriage. At nineteen years of age he
entered the service of the Carnegie Company as a
"stake driver." He gradually rose till he became
President of the Bethlehem Steel Company. He is
said to have spent large sums on educational institutions,
a fact that indicates that he recognises the value of
education for others.

On the other hand, Mr. Hoover, the Food Controller,
took his degree in geology at Stanford University. But
one of his fellow students has informed me that, before
doing so, he showed business capacity in starting a
laundry which turned out to be a great success. Therefore Mr. Hoover is not an instance of a man beginning
as an expert and afterwards developing business capacity
but the reverse.

The facts brought forward in this chapter supply further evidence that the act of forgetting is a necessary prelude for putting data at the disposal of the subconscious mind for the purpose of subconscious judgment. This is the explanation of Montaigne's conclusion that excellent memories accompany weak judgments. This is the reason why the business instinct is badly developed among the more erudite products of our universities. Hence also we find among experts that those with best memories have least originality. Hence the common experience that, on studying a new subject, the better kind of original ideas about it only occur to us after the details are more or less forgotten. The original ideas that come to us while we are actually studying the subject are of the nature of explanations made up on the spur of the moment. Such explanations have little value. They represent the critical faculty at its worst.

CHAPTER VIII

Lord Kelvin and the Atlantic Cable—Business men needing help in dealing with Inventors—Need of two kinds of experts.

A government official once said in the House of Commons that he knew of many commercial concerns which had been ruined by having highly gifted scientific men on their boards. This statement raises the question whether the scientist is in his right position on the board of a commercial company. The story of Lord Kelvin's connection with commercial companies will be found to furnish evidence bearing on this point.

Lord Kelvin (he was then Professor Thomson) was one of the directors of the first company for laying a cable across the Atlantic. Mr. Whitehouse, a retired medical man, and in electrical matters little better than a quack, was appointed electrician to the company. The consequences of this arrangement were disastrous. The directors, being business men, naturally were guided by their electrician who spoke to them with authority because of his official post. Lord Kelvin spoke to them with no such authority but with reasoned arguments. What the company wanted or rather needed from Lord Kelvin was not his reasoning or his reasons. They needed his conclusions. Had he been a consulting expert to the company, the directors would have been more likely to accept his conclusions than was the case when he took part in their deliberations.

The actual history of the cable was as follows : The cable was laid. A few messages were sent through it with difficulty and then after a few days it ceased to work. Too late the directors discovered that the cable had been ruined by the strong currents that had been employed by their electrician against the advice of Lord Kelvin.

The directors dismissed Mr. Whitehouse, and Lord Kelvin " with an excess of generosity asked the Board to condone Whitehouse's errors of judgment." Such generosity was obviously quite incompatible with good business and suggests that Lord Kelvin was lacking in the business instinct. The directors replied to him as follows :—

" Mr. Whitehouse has been engaged some 18 months in investigations, which have cost some £12,000 to this company, so that he has been in a position to avail himself of every resource that would tend to accomplish the objects on which he was at work, and now when we have laid our cable and the whole world is looking on with impatience to realise some results from our success, we are, after all, only saved from being a laughing stock because the Directors are fortunate enough to have an illustrious colleague who has devoted his mind to this subject, and whose inventions produced *in his own study* at *small expense*—and from his own *resources* are available to supersede the useless portions of apparatus prepared at great labour and enormous cost for this special occasion."

This was in 1858. Some years later, in 1865, the project was revived. Lord Kelvin was again employed by the company, but this time as a consulting expert. The directors listened to his advice, used his transmitting and receiving instruments, and the cable was a success. With later cable companies Lord Kelvin was also in his proper position as consulting electrician and not as a director, so far as can be gathered from his biography.*

In considering the question whether experts should follow Lord Kelvin's example and become consulting experts to commercial companies, or whether, on the other hand, they should become directors, it must be borne in mind that a business man is likely to give more weight to a conclusion for which he has paid than he will to a long reasoned argument that he is incapable of appreciating. Further, a business man is accustomed to arrive at decisions by acts of his subconscious judgment for which he is unable to give reasons that would satisfy his expert colleague. The latter's reasoning power will often connote a capacity for talking against which the business man may be helpless and by which he may be convinced " against his better judgment," or, if this does not happen, by which valuable time may be wasted.

Some years ago there existed a commercial company

---

* A more detailed account will be found in *Life of Lord Kelvin*, by Sylvanus P. Thompson (Macmillan & Co., 1910).

the directors of which were all experts. They paid no dividends. Before their final dissolution they attracted attention by getting involved in a lawsuit in which the evidence showed that they suffered from a singular incapacity for getting things done. Information came to me from two sources to the effect that they were apt to be guided by vague suspicions based on long drawn out reasoning on occasions when data for such reasoning were insufficient and where ordinary business men would have arrived at once at common-sense decisions with the help of their subconscious judgments.

Apropos of a discussion as to the governing of London University, Professor Huxley wrote : " As for a government by professors only, the fact of their being specialists is against them. Most of them are broad-minded, practical men ; some are good administrators. But, unfortunately, there is among them, as in other professions, a fair sprinkling of one-idea'd fanatics, ignorant of the commonest conventions of official relation, and content with nothing if they cannot get everything their own way. It is these persons who, with the very highest and purest intentions, would ruin any administrative body unless they were counterpoised by non-professional common-sense members of recognised weight and authority in the conduct of affairs."*

Thus in Professor Huxley's opinion, the " one-idea'd fanatics " could be better counterpoised by "common-sense members " than by professors though most of

---

* *Life and Letters of Thomas Henry Huxley*, by Leonard Huxley (Macmillan & Co., 1908), Vol. III., p. 233.

them are broad-minded practical men and some are good administrators. It may be surmised that " common-sense members " would be less ready than the professors to listen to the formal reasoning on which the fanatics would inevitably depend.

Experts do not always realise what is wanted in a commercial affair. A speaker in a discussion on industrial chemists, in 1917, stated that " the commercial training of the chemist was a very difficult subject, because there was the jealousy of the commercial man to deal with. The average commercial man learnt by association with the firm and learnt very easily indeed. The wonderful principles of finance were very simple, and any man with a chemical training would easily learn them."

This statement lends itself to criticism. Why should the expert be troubled by the jealousy of the commercial man ? It is possible that the appearance of jealousy is the result of the business man's incapacity for giving reasons for his common-sense decisions that would satisfy the logical mind of the expert.

The above speaker seems to hold the very questionable belief that business ability is something that can be learnt out of books. There is no evidence at all that those intuitional powers of the mind that comprise the business instinct can be acquired in this way. On the contrary the business instinct seems to develop most readily in those whose heads are least filled with book learning and who often have a most surprising power of forgetting.

The business instinct and the power of scientific reasoning are so opposed to each other in mental method, and so generally found in separate heads that it is reasonable to suspect that the development of one hinders the development of the other.

The above considerations probably apply justly to instances where it is desired to make a continued application of some known scientific discovery, but they fail to prove that the combination of business instinct and ignorance is sufficient where new processes or methods are involved.

For instance, as has been stated above, ill-educated Mahomedan merchants in India, in certain businesses are superior to members of better educated communities. The Mahomedans appear to be less successful in those lines of business that make demands on intelligence, knowledge and capacity for progress rather than they do on the instinctive powers of the mind. To test this point two lists were compiled by me of occupations of merchants in Bombay. One was of those demanding knowledge and enterprise. The other was of occupations that make more demand on the business instinct than on knowledge. The first list contained accountants, architects, surveyors, auctioneers, bankers, billiard table makers, booksellers and publishers, brokers, carbonic acid gas dealers, chemists and druggists, cinematograph importers, clearing and forwarding agents, coach builders, decorators, gramophone dealers, jewellers, gold and silver smiths, machinery importers, opticians, photographers, photographic material dealers, provision merchants and sewing machine dealers. The second list comprised bookbinders, boot and shoe makers, carpet dealers, cotton and woollen merchants, glassware merchants, hardware dealers, horse importers, hosiery merchants, paint and colour dealers, paper merchants, perfumers, woollen goods dealers, saddlers and harness makers, stationers, sugar merchants, tailors, dressmakers and outfitters, tanneries and hide merchants, and timber merchants. The first list included 1,154 firms of which 50, or four per cent., had Mahomedan names. The second list comprised 1,152 firms of which 483, or forty-two per cent., had Mahomedan names. Thus the Mahomedans in Bombay figure far more largely in occupations dealing with staple products and in products which have been imported for many years than they do in occupations of more recent origin or that demand new or special knowledge.

Some years ago the whole of the trade in matches in Calcutta was reputed to be in the hands of one Mahomedan merchant. He was said to sell his matches at cost price and to make his profit on the packing cases. The mental equipment of this merchant, though ample for his business, would, no doubt, be entirely insufficient for a maker of chemicals who must continually be on the look out for improved processes owing to the advances of science. In the making of aniline dyes, not only are new dyes being discovered but the users of the dyes have sometimes to be educated in their use. Whether a new dye should be made or an existing dye dropped will depend on many factors whose value can only be properly appreciated by experts ; for instance, it will depend, not only on the availability of new raw materials but also on the possibility of utilising bye products in other branches of the factory, etc.

The boards of German dye manufacturing companies include men of scientific training and who have much practical knowledge of chemistry. It does not follow that any expert distinguished for his discoveries in pure science is necessarily in his right place on the board of a commercial company that deals with some scientific product. The German chemist who finds himself on the board of such a company is a man who has had many years experience of commercial work and who has been selected from a large number of commercial chemists.

An account of the method of producing a German commercial chemist has been given by Dr. M. O. Forster.* He says that it is amply proved by experience at the large German chemical factories that much time is required to discover a man's capacities, that " though ample promise may be given at the age of 30, full development is not usually reached before 40 and in many cases even later. If then a factory staff of 50 chemists, recruited at 22 or thereabouts, be allowed to develop under the influence of factory surroundings and requirements, there will prevail throughout the organisation an interchange of thought and outlook

---

* *Journal of the Society of Chemical Industry*, July 31st, 1915, Vol. XXXIV, p. 760.

contributing to the highest degree of chemical development along the lines of individual temperament. The legal-minded man will gravitate towards the factory patent office, the bookworm towards the library. The skilful analyst will become the indispensable and time-saving support of the discoverer who will ransack raw and waste materials assisted by the man who has found his calling to be preparation. . . The whole point is that at 22, one is only dimly conscious of being either legal-minded, a bookworm, an analyst, a discoverer, a preparator, a mechanician, or a human person, and that given the necessary chemical rudiments, a plunge into the above mentioned system is the best way for a young chemist to classify himself." Thus, according to this description, the German commercial chemist is expected to gravitate towards the particular branch of the work for which he finds himself best fitted. The process of education seems to be a process of finding out what he likes best and giving him opportunities of doing it. As we shall see later, such a method lacks the kind of discipline necessary for developing the intuitional powers of the mind. One would anticipate that a man so educated would be well capable of using his conscious reason in choosing which of several lines of research to follow but to lack the instinctive power of making such a choice, a power to which the success of great scientific discoverers is frequently attributed. Under the strain of war also, German chemists appear to have been wanting in initiative and adaptability.* As has

---

* *Journal of the Chemical Society*, April, 1919, p. 402.

already been stated the success of German chemical concerns is more due to their having good things to sell than to the possession of real business capacity.

An occasion on which a business man requires the help of formal reason rather than of common sense is when he is dealing with new inventions. Supposing an inventor comes to a business man with proposals for a new process or a new invention and invites the business man to finance the undertaking, then there can be no doubt that in such an eventuality the use of such reason is demanded. The reasoning power of the inventor will inevitably be prejudiced in favour of his invention. The reasoning power of the business man will be handicapped by his probable lack of the necessary technical knowledge. What is required is for the business man to get independent advice from an expert. Not every expert is suitable. He must get an expert who is not too anxious to display his own knowledge. He must, if possible, get an expert who is accustomed to give decisions as to the value of the inventions of others. If the business man engages an expert who lacks such qualifications, he may get something of the nature of carping criticism rather than reasoned judgment. Several such instances are known to me. For instance, on my once suggesting that a certain research might lead to important results, my idea was submitted to an expert in the subject who simply pulverised my suggestion. It afterwards came to my knowledge that this expert, in a book he had written, had himself advocated the very same idea that he now criticised so violently. He had forgotten what he had written and his judgment perhaps was vitiated by the appearance of an interloper on his preserves.

In Germany the inventor of a new process does not find it necessary to persuade a business man to promote a company to develop his invention. He applies to one of the banks that undertake this kind of work. The bank employs a staff of experts who investigate the whole subject. Not only are there experts for the scientific and technical aspects of the matter, but also there are special experts who report on such subjects as " costing," the supply of raw materials and the probable demand. No attractive prospectus is issued. No exaggerated statements are made to influence an unwilling public. No expenses are incurred in publicly promoting a company or underwriting its shares. The bank itself advances the money if it is satisfied with the reports of its experts. It was in this way that capital was obtained for the first manufactories for the fixation of atmospheric nitrogen, a matter of the greatest commercial importance. Had it not been for this industry, Germany would have run short of explosives at a very early stage of the great war.

Thus in commercial matters, as in law, there is a need for two kinds of experts : one whose qualifications should be skill and originality and whose work it is to make discoveries : the other, for whom age and experience are more important than originality, whose business it should be to give judicial opinions on discoveries submitted for consideration. In a later chapter examples will be related of men of business falling victims to swindlers simply because, in scientific matters, they preferred to trust their own reason rather than the reason of an independent expert.

NOTE.

In America, before the war, German dyes had a well-deserved reputation and success. Not content with this, and with their strange tendency towards the crooked and the immoral, the agents of the German dye companies developed an astonishing system of commercial immorality. For instance, their agents started a laboratory for a research for discovering chemicals that, if put surreptitiously into dye vats, would result in bad dyeing. The purpose of this was to get a means of discrediting rival dyes. Their own dyes were sold adulterated to different degrees and under different names to different customers, and a very complicated system of accounts had to be maintained to ensure that each dyer's foreman received the right amount of graft. The system was a product of short-sighted reason rather than of common sense. A business man has described it to me as childish. The Germans overlooked the fact that such a system was bound to have a demoralising effect on their employees and also that it was very likely to be found out. This happened, with resulting scandal and loss of trade. One American dye-works, by eliminating graft, reduced its yearly expenditure on dyestuffs from 265,000 to 125,000 dollars. My authority for these statements is an article by H. C. Burr on " German business methods in the United States," *Quarterly Review*, July, 1916, p. 16.

CHAPTER IX

EXPERTS AS BUSINESS MEN

Lord Kelvin's success in exploiting his inventions—His partnership with engineers—Edison—Agassiz and other experts
successful in business—Inventors.

The expert has been described, in the preceding
chapters, as having a different mental outfit from that
of the successful man of business. The expert depends
mainly on formal logical processes. The business man
depends mainly on rapid common-sense decisions.

It may be objected to this description that instances
are known of experts being successful in business. It
is necessary therefore to examine these alleged cases.

Lord Kelvin is known to have made a great deal of
money by his inventions. But on reading his life, it is
clear that he was successful in this respect only when
he was in partnership with practical men. For example,
as regards his patents, he was in partnership with
Varley, an electrician, and Fleeming Jenkin, an engineer.
The story of the best known of his patents is as follows :

When the first Atlantic cable was laid, it was found
that, for some abstruse reasons whose nature was discovered by Lord Kelvin, extremely feeble currents of
electricity had to be employed. At first the only way
of detecting these currents was by means of Lord Kelvin's
" mirror galvanometer." The current from the cable

was passed into this instrument and caused oscillations of a small magnet. A minute mirror was attached to the magnet and served to reflect a beam of light on to a screen. The movements of the spot of light thus produced represented telegraphic signals which could be interpreted by a skilled observer. The spot of light had to be watched constantly day and night—a very fatiguing duty. Such was the sensitiveness of the instrument that the spot of light was easily deflected by a current received through the whole length of the cable from a battery made of a lady's thimble, a small piece of zinc and a few drops of dilute acid. It would seem an insoluble problem to get sufficient power, out of such feeble currents, to move a pen which could write down the signals on a moving ribbon of paper. But this problem Lord Kelvin solved with his marvellously ingenious instrument the "siphon recorder." Its use by the companies was inevitable. It was only after they had agreed to pay royalty on his previous instrument, the mirror galvanometer, that he brought out the siphon recorder. He charged the companies £1,000 a year for permission to use it. Thenceforward every company that laid down a cable had to pay Lord Kelvin £1,000 a year for using his instrument.

From the point of view of business Lord Kelvin had a very easy furrow to hoe. Business acumen was needed, not by Lord Kelvin, but rather by the promoters of the companies who had to calculate whether the traffic would indemnify them for the expense incurred in paying royalties and laying the cables.

It is recorded that, in 1881, Lord Kelvin and several
of his friends spent some time in attempting to start a
company to exploit the Faure accumulator. The agent
of the French patentees is said to have had a marvellous
genius for drafting prospectuses. " The negotiations
lasted through August, as one by one withdrew from
taking part in so formidable a venture ; but it was not
till some weeks later that Sir William (afterwards Lord
Kelvin) was brought to realise the very unsatisfactory
position ; and he too withdrew—a heavy loser by the
affair—from all association with the venture, though he
wished the invention success."*

The friends of Lord Kelvin showed the business
instinct by withdrawing from the affair in time. The
same cannot be said of Lord Kelvin. His wishing the
invention success shows a bias which, however commendable from his point of view, cannot be described as good
for business.

Edison has made large sums of money by his inventions. He lacked the ordinary education of an expert.
As a child he was " rather wanting in ordinary acumen "
but was highly inquisitive and had an extraordinarily
retentive memory. He had three months schooling
only and afterwards was taught by his mother who was
well-informed and ambitious. He early showed a taste
for experiment, for finding out things for himself rather
than for learning them from others. After some of his
discoveries had made him famous, he got an oppor-

---

* *Life of Lord Kelvin*, by Silvanus P. Thompson, pp. 575, 623,
650 and 770.

tunity of experimenting with 2,000 miles of telegraph cable coiled up in a tank. He says about this : " I sent a single dot, which should have been recorded upon my automatic paper by a mark about one thirty-second of an inch long. Instead of that it was twenty-seven feet long. If ever I had any conceit it vanished from my boots up. What I did not know at the time was that a coiled cable, owing to induction, was infinitely worse than when laid out straight." It is remarkable that a man who had discovered quadruplex telegraphy did not know a fact of this nature.

Thus, at first sight, Edison appears to offer an instance of an expert having business capacity. The first explanation that occurred to me was that he was an inventor rather than a true scientific expert. But a very different view of the matter has been expressed by Mr. Ford of automobile fame. He says : " Edison is easily the world's greatest scientist. I am not sure that he is not also the world's worst business man. He knows almost nothing of business."* As regards business capacity, at all events, Mr. Ford's opinion may be safely accepted.

Therefore, as with the German aniline dye manufacturers, as also with Lord Kelvin, Edison's success in money making appears rather to be due to his having good things to sell than to the possession of real business instinct.

The story told of the younger Agassiz is that he wished

* *My Life and Work by Henry Ford* (London, Heinemann, 1922). p. 235.

to follow in his father's footsteps and devote his life to zoology.   To be able to do so, money was required. He resolved to begin by making it.   He took his degree at Harvard in 1855 and afterwards studied engineering and chemistry.   Then he became an assistant in the United States Coast Survey.   His next move was to become Superintendant of the Calumet and Hecla Copper Mine.   This mine did not conform to the classical description in being a hole in the ground with a fool at the bottom and a knave at the top, as it turned out to be a considerable source of profit.   It was only after he had made money in this way that Agassiz developed into an expert in zoological subjects.

Benjamin Franklin (1706-1790), the American diplomatist and scientist, had only two years of school life. At the age of ten he was apprenticed to a tallow chandler. Later he became a printer.   It was only after this that he developed scientific aptitudes.   In 1737 he published a paper on the causes of earthquakes.   In 1749 he discovered the lightning conductor.   He carried out his celebrated experiment of getting electricity from a kite-string in 1752.   A singular example of the utility of science is the fact that this experiment, by proving that thunder and lightning were due to natural causes, dealt a blow against the then prevalent belief that storms were due to witchcraft and thus indirectly helped to put a stop to the persecution of witches.

Count Rumford (1753-1814), an American, was apprenticed to a store-keeper at the age of thirteen.   In his spare time he carried out chemical and mechanical experiments. He was precocious in mathematics and at the age of fourteen he calculated a solar eclipse within four seconds of accuracy. He became an administrator and only at a later date showed scientific originality. He published his discovery that heat is a mode of motion in 1798.

Sir Joseph Whitworth (1813-1887), the engineer, well known for his work in introducing accurate methods into the machine shop, left school at the age of fourteen. He then became a cotton spinner and at eighteen worked under a machine-manufacturer. In 1840 he published his first scientific paper. It dealt with true planes.

Sir Henry Bessemer (1813-1898) was the discoverer of an improved method of making steel. After completing his education he started a steel works. He discovered his improved methods of manufacture in 1856.

Sir William Armstrong (1800-1900), the engineer, was a solicitor from 1833 to 1847. In 1841 he published a paper on electricity produced by effluent steam.

Sir William Huggins (1824-1910) was a wealthy brewer who took up astronomy as a hobby and afterwards became distinguished in that science.

Sir Andrew Noble (1832-1915) entered the Royal Artillery in 1849. In 1857 he became secretary to the Royal Artillery Institution. He became known as an expert in explosives and in 1859 joined the Elswick works.

Lord Avebury (1832-1913) was sent to Eton in 1845 and in 1848 joined his father's bank. In 1856 be became partner. It was after this that he began to show scientific originality. In 1865 he published his book on " *Prehistoric Times,*" in 1870 a book on " *The Origin of Civilisation,*" and in 1873 another on the *Origin and Metamorphoses of Insects.* His father, Sir John Lubbock, was a banker who published papers dealing with mathematical subjects.

Thus in all the above instances of experts of business or administrative ability, there is not one in which the expert began his life with an expert's education or bent of mind. In every case, before he showed scientific originality, he had been in a position in which there was a demand for the employment of the intuitional powers of the mind rather than for the pure formal reasoning that is needed by the expert in scientific research.

During the war it occasionally happened that experts were called on to undertake administrative work and did so with success. It is an interesting question whether, while doing such work, they retained their expert frame of mind. One instance has been quoted in which, after doing administrative work, a geological expert had forgotten elementary facts of geology. An instance has been related to me in which an expert in chemistry obtained an administrative post and afterwards entered a business in which he appears to have done well. He asserts he has completely forgotten all his scientific knowledge.

K

CHAPTER X

Doubling gold—Destroying a man by magic—Forging of currency notes—Trick with copper coins—A Thug story—Inventors.

" A lady palmist and astrologer is willing to accord interviews to business men and speculators." So runs an advertisement in a daily paper. The question arises why is it that business men, who are usually cautious in their affairs, should sometimes be ready to accept the statements of a lady astrologer or be taken in by all kinds of swindlers. An instance is known to me of the head of a large commercial firm losing all his ready money by means of the three card trick during a railway journey. According to a newspaper account, a few years ago, a swindler once persuaded some business men that he could manufacture diamonds. These business men, instead of calling in expert advice, themselves tried to judge the value of the invention and, for some time, were taken in by diamonds that had been introduced into the apparatus by sleight of hand.

Sir Robert Anderson tells a story of a London house, " whose name is in high repute in all the capitals of Europe," being taken in by a swindler who professed to have the power of increasing gold. Whatever amount of gold was given to him, he had, he said, the power of doubling its quantity. The firm, instead of getting an independent expert to investigate the matter, thought that they themselves were capable of estimating the value of a supposedly scientific experiment and offered the swindler £100 for the purpose. He declined this paltry sum as entailing mere waste of time. At length the firm put up £20,000 and took a house especially for the experiment, in Leman Street, Whitechapel. The conditions demanded by the swindler were (1) that no one else should be allowed to enter the laboratory and (2) that he should be rigorously searched every time he went out. He had a gold-headed walking stick. The members of the firm no doubt thought this gold-headed walking stick was in keeping with the part. This was unfortunate for them as it was hollow. The swindler used the hollow space to remove the sovereigns, carrying away as many as it would hold at each visit. When they had all been abstracted in this way, he wrote to the firm explaining what he had done and daring them to report the matter to the police.*

To understand how business men, men of common sense, can be deceived by such methods we shall find some help in studying various forms of the confidence trick. Let us consider some examples.

A stranger in Bombay, who may be referred to as the dupe, while walking in the street, happened to make the acquaintance of a man who may be described as Villain No. 1. They went into a restaurant together

* *The Lighter Side of my Official Life*, by Sir Robert Anderson (Hodder and Stoughton, London, 1910).

and called for coffee. Presently Villain No. 1 pointed out a man sitting at the other side of the room, who, he said, was a remarkable magician. He had such powerful incantations that, by their means, he could destroy a man who was miles away. The magician was Villain No. 2. No. 1 had scarcely finished his description when an acquaintance (No. 3) arrived and sat down by them. They changed the subject and began to talk of trivial matters. Suddenly No. 3 saw walking at the opposite side of the road a man whom he described to them as being a rich Mahomedan merchant that he knew slightly. This supposed merchant was Villain No. 4. This merchant, said No. 3, had recently had a quarrel with a man named Allah Buksh. Such was his anger and enmity that he was ready to pay a reward of five thousand rupees to anybody who would kill Allah Buksh. Villain No. 1 at once winked to the dupe and, hastily taking leave of No. 3, the two left the restaurant together. " Here is a chance," said he to the dupe, " of our making our fortunes. Let us speak to the merchant, make terms with him and then bring the magician to his house." The dupe consented. He had no time to think as they were hurrying along the road. They spoke to the merchant, who fired up on hearing the name of Allah Buksh, and willingly consented to the plan of employing the magician. No. 1 and the dupe went back to the restaurant, explained matters to the magician and brought him to the merchant's house. The incantations were duly performed and then No. 1 and the dupe went out for a walk probably to find out whether anything had happened to Allah Buksh. Presently they met a stranger who was crying bitterly. They stopped to ask him the cause of his grief. He replied that his dearest friend Allah Buksh was walking along the street a few minutes ago, apparently in the best of health, when he suddenly staggered and fell down dead. After expressing sympathy with the stranger (Villain No. 5) they returned to the house of the supposed merchant with what the dupe regarded as perfectly independent evidence of the success of the incantations. They began to claim the reward when, without warning, the magician fell down seized with a very alarming fit. No. 1 thereupon explained to the dupe and the merchant that the magician was liable to such seizures after performing his magical rites and that the only remedy was to wait till he was a little better and then to take him to the Jain temple at the end of Abdur Rahman Street. The magician soon showed signs of improvement and they all went out together. Unfortunately, when on their way to the temple, they were arrested by a policeman on a charge of murder of a man named Allah Buksh. The dupe thus received a further and most unwelcome proof of the efficacy of the incantations. While on their way to the police station, No, 1 suggested to the dupe that, as their guilt was known, their only chance was to bribe the policeman to let them go. There was no great difficulty in doing this, as the policeman was Villain No. 6. The dupe gave up all the money in his possession. As soon as they were free, the villain No. 1

pointed out that they were still liable to arrest and that they must fly. This they did, in different directions, leaving the dupe slowly to awake from his dream of wealth and to realise that he had been swindled.

The use of photography in the bogus forging of currency notes appears to be a practical application of science peculiar to India. The stock-in-trade of a professor of this art was once sent to me for examination. A number of bottles of essences and coloured pigments and packets of powders were contained in a box about ten inches long, six inches wide and about six inches deep. Each of the edges of the box was strengthened with a few short strips of sheet brass. On raising the lid a small shelf about an inch wide was found running along the length of the top of the box on the side nearest the hinges. The purpose of this shelf was to conceal a false bottom. This false bottom normally was kept standing up against the rear side of the box. It was held in position by a catch. On pressing one of the brass strips on the outside of the box the catch releases the false bottom, allowing it to full down and hide the true bottom of the box. The *modus operandi* was as follows :

The swindler represents to the dupe that he has the power of duplicating currency notes. The bottles and powders are merely for show. The swindler takes a ten rupee currency note, places it on a piece of photographic sensitive paper and covers it with a sheet of glass. It is exposed for a few minutes to the sun. On raising the glass, an impression of the currency note is found on the sensitive paper. This is shown to the dupe as the first stage in the process. The dupe is then asked to look into the box to satisfy himself that it is empty. The inside of the box is black in colour, an arrangement that helps to conceal the false bottom. The dupe being convinced that there is nothing in the box is asked to put into it the half-made currency note. This he does and then closes the lid. The swindler then performs his incantations. Then, pointing out that he has not touched the note or the box at all, he picks up the latter and, in so doing, presses the secret spring. The false bottom falls down thereby concealing the half-made note and liberating a real rurrency note that had been concealed behind it. He hands the box to the dupe and asks him to open it. The dupe does so and finds the real currency note. Without giving him time to think, the swindler sends him off to the bazaar to buy some tobacco and to change the note so as to get a proof that the note is good currency. When the dupe comes back, the swindler offers, as a favour, or, more probably for some consideration, to duplicate a note for a thousand rupees. The dupe produces such a note. This time the procedure is different. The photographic impression is made as before and the swindler pretends to tie this up in a parcel with the real currency note. But he abstracts the latter by sleight of hand. The parcel is buried in the ground. The swindler performs his incantations and orders that the parcel should only be dug up after an interval of three days as otherwise the magic will not work. The swindler then departs having a three days' start. Probably he has a longer start, for, after the dupe discovers he has been cheated, he may hesitate a little before admitting to the police that he was concerned in an attempted forgery of currency notes.

When the anarchist agitation began in India some years ago, a gang of swindlers made use of it in a very unexpected way. They arrived at Delhi and began buying up all the copper coins of a particular issue. The price began to go up. Soon they were giving three or four annas for a half anna coin. Much interest was aroused. Everyone was trying to find out why these coins were wanted. At last when the price had risen to seven or eight annas, one of the confederates did divulge the secret under the strictest seal of confidence. The anarchists in Calcutta, he said, wishing to embarrass the Government, had got into the Mint one night and dropped some plates of gold they found there into a pot of melted copper. It was from this copper that the 1906 issue of copper coins had been made. Each coin was worth therefore several rupees. Gradually the secret got out. Some strangers arrived, who were confederates and who had a large supply of these coins. Everybody was soon buying them right and left and the price rose to between fifteen and twenty annas. The original buyers, who had bought at three or four annas now quietly sold out at the higher rate. They then vanished and the half anna coin somewhat rapidly returned to its normal rate of exchange.

The dropped trinket trick is well known in England.

A trinket which appears to be of gold is picked up by the dupe and returned to the swindler who, to prove his gratitude, sells it to him at a very low price. The dupe afterwards finds that it is made of brass. In a variant of this trick found in India, the dropped trinket is a bracelet. A pair of swindlers, after meeting the dupe, find the bracelet lying on the ground. Presently they meet a stranger in bitter grief who explains that he has lost a gold bracelet worth thirty rupees. The dupe thus obtains an impartial estimate of its value. Having parted from the stranger, they soon come to cross roads where, as they are going different ways, the dupe is persuaded to take the bracelet and pay the two swindlers their share of it in cash. Naturally on trying to sell the bracelet the dupe learns that it is made of brass.

A clue to the psychological basis of these tricks is yielded by an old Thug story. The case is of interest because two failures preceded the success. An Indian who had a great reputation for personal courage was travelling through a district infested by Thugs. A party of these robbers resolved to murder him. Knowing his route they went on in front and allowed him to overtake some of their party. They pretended to be a set of poor people and implored his protection. Their intended victim was suspicious and drove them away. Making a detour they again got in front. Again he overtook them and found them disguised as rich Hindu merchants. They said they had much money with them : they were afraid of Thugs and would willingly pay for his protection. Again the victim was suspicious and refused to travel with them. Again they went on ahead. He again overtook them and found them disguised as Mahomedan soldiers. One was lying on the ground wrapped in a sheet. A grave was dug beside the supposed body. They told their victim that one of their comrades had died. They wished to bury him, but being too ignorant to offer up prayers in accordance with custom, they implored his help. The grief of these poor ignorant soldiers aroused the pity of their victim. He dismounted, put down his weapons and knelt in prayer. At once the strangling handkerchief was round his neck. In a few moments he was dead ; his valuables were stolen and he was rapidly buried in the grave that had already been prepared.

The point of importance in this story is that the victim only lost his caution when his emotions were aroused.

This is the psychological basis of the confidence trick. The swindler vitiates the judgment of his dupe by playing on his emotions. In each of the tricks above described, the success of the swindler was due to his offering the dupe the prospect of much gain with little trouble or risk. The desire for gain, no doubt, underlies every legitimate commercial transaction but it is usually balanced by the prospect of having to work to achieve success and also by the risk of losing one's time or one's money. In confidence tricks the desire for gain is not properly balanced, partly because the scheme is unexpected, partly because gain is offered without risk, and partly because there is no prospect of hard work.

This is an example of the general rule that it is not the emotion but the unbalanced emotion that vitiates judgment. Any get-rich-quick scheme that offers us other people's money without risk or without our having to work for it, should be regarded with suspicion, not because it is necessarily bad, but because—from its nature—it handicaps our reason and puts us mentally in the position of the victims of the confidence trick.

Our reliance on this explanation of confidence tricks will be increased if examples of a different nature can be quoted in which prospect of gain does harm to judgment. Let us consider the case of inventors.

Inventors have the common reputation of being lacking in business ability. For instance, an inventor once proposed to a manufacturing company that they should exploit a secret process that he had discovered. An agreement was drawn up in which he undertook to explain the process in return for a royalty. A day was appointed for its signature and the inventor duly arrived. Then some trivial reason transpired for which it was necessary to defer signing the agreement. This would be done, it was said, on the following day. In the meantime the inventor, unfortunately for him, was induced to divulge his process. The signature is still wanting and the inventor has been defrauded of his profits.

In another instance the inventor was not satisfied with the terms of a proposed agreement. The business men with whom he was dealing thereupon began to play on his emotions. They invited him to dinner and treated him, as he said, with extreme kindness. What specially impressed him was, as he explained to his friends, that they had promised him various advantages and profits over and above those mentioned in the agreement. His friends, whose emotions had not been played on, were able to give him some salutary advice.

The inventor's ideal is fifty per cent. of the profits, he furnishing the brains and the other man the capital. On my once making a suggestion to this effect—but in other words—to a business man, about some mechanical contrivance, he at once fell in with the idea. It was always well in such cases, he explained, to have the agreement in black and white, so we drew one up and signed it on the spot. My idea of what it should contain was quite clear, but, at the time, something blinded my judgment as to what it did contain. The invention came to nothing but, some years later, on reading the agreement, it was found by me to contain a statement that the cost of patenting should not exceed a certain amount. There was not a word as to who should defray this cost.

In each of these instances the inventor's work was done. He had made his invention and all he had to do was to wait for his reward. He had the prospect of gain without having to work for it and, as with the dupes of the confidence trick, his common sense was in default.

An author who has finished writing a book is in a similar position. But long experience has taught authors that it is, in many cases at least, advisable for them to employ literary agents to conclude their agreements with publishers. Inventors have need of similar assistance. Without it, both authors and inventors are liable, to their detriment, to illustrate the rule that an unbalanced desire vitiates judgment.

CHAPTER XI

THE MENTAL LIMITATIONS OF THE GLOBE-TROTTER

Instances of globe-trotters' defective judgment—Mr. H. G. Wells
in Russia—Inexperienced commercial travellers—Influence
of strange surroundings on memory—Advantages of travelling in enlarging basis of experience.

In this chapter the familiar term " globe-trotter "
will be used to designate those travellers whose judgment appears to be affected by the strangeness of their
surroundings.

Many years ago a member of Parliament was travelling
in India at a time when a certain part of the country was
affected by famine.   By a very remarkable organisation,
government was cheaply and efficiently giving daily
relief to some six million people.   This merely aroused
the visitor's indignation.   He wanted government to
move the distressed population to the banks of the river
Indus, then and at once, oblivious of all the difficulties
that might accompany the transport of six million
people and finding food for them till they had raised
their crops in their new environment.

A cultivated American gentleman, when on his way
back after sunset from some sight-seeing in Agra, noticed
a light on the opposite bank of the river.   " What is
that ? " said he to me.   " That," I replied, " is an
electric light on the top of a flour mill belonging to Messrs.

John and Company. It is thirty-two candle power."
" Indeed it isn't," said he, " it is the light on the top of
a Parsee fire temple." As a matter of fact there are
no Parsee fire temples within many hundred miles of
Agra.

An Australian gentleman travelling on a P. & O.
steamer, once told me that he was interested in emigrants and had a good deal to do with helping them on
their arrival in Australia. On my asking him how
long after their arrival these emigrants showed lack of
common sense, he said with surprise, " How do you
know they do? Have you ever been in Australia? " My
reply was to the effect that my question was due to my
study of the natural history of globe-trotters in other
places than in Australia. He told me that freshly
arrived emigrants do as a fact often show a conspicuous
lack of judgment and that this lack of judgment generally
lasts for about a year. He told me also of an American
gentleman who had had exactly the same experience
of emigrants in New York.

It might be suggested that such instances of lack of
judgment merely prove that the travellers in question
were stupid people and that they probably would say
equally stupid things when at home. This suggestion,
however, does not appear to be correct. Lack of judgment when travelling may be shown by persons of high
ability.

For instance, when plague broke out in Bombay in
1896, many distinguished scientists came from Europe
to investigate the disease. For the time being they

were globe-trotters and their reports perhaps showed less scientific acumen than might have been expected. One of these scientists, shortly after his arrival, was found to be suffering from a fixed idea that plague was due to lack of ventilation. He had himself seen that plague-infected houses were ill-ventilated and was unduly impressed with the value of his observation. He was on a commission before which I gave evidence. " Dr. Hankin," he said, " I hear that you do not think that lack of ventilation is the sole cause of plague. Please give us a reason." My reply was to the effect that " When plague broke out in Hardwar, monkeys were affected in far greater proportion than human beings, though these monkeys never go into unventilated places." After a whispered remark from a member of the commission whose sense of humour was well-developed, he asked me " How do you know that monkeys would not have suffered still more severely if they had gone into insanitary places ? " My answer was, " Government realising the danger, had these monkeys caught, put in cages and liberated a hundred miles away in the jungle. While in the cages, which were very over-crowded and quite insanitary, not a single monkey suffered from plague." This reply elicited the remark, " That will do, Dr. Hankin, I don't believe you know anything at all about it."*

The late Sir Lauder Brunton demurred on my telling

---

* It was impossible for Government to kill these monkeys as they are regarded as sacred by the inhabitants of Hardwar. As my questioner is no longer living the above story may be told without risk of hurting anyone's feelings.

him that in my opinion a man was mentally handicapped when in strange surroundings. He told me he had once come to India to carry out a certain research. He found out so much in that time, he said, that, when he got home, it took him two years to write out an account of his discoveries. His receptive powers were not diminished and perhaps were increased while he was in India. But his power of performing an act of judgment on the facts discovered was only shown, and perhaps was only available when he had returned home and ceased to be a globe-trotter.

There is even room for the suspicion that a man of such exceptional ability as Mr. H. G. Wells was suffering from similar disabilities during a visit paid by him to Russia in 1920. Before his arrival he anticipated that some attempt might be made to deceive him as to the true facts of the case. He was therefore forewarned. He says :

" The guide and interpreter assigned to assist us was a lady I had met in Russia in 1914, the niece of a former Russian Ambassador to London. She was educated at Newnham, she had been imprisoned five times by the Bolshevist Government, she is not allowed to leave Petersburg because of an attempt to cross the frontier to her children in Esthonia, and she was, therefore, the last person likely to hoodwink us."

There seems to be something wrong with this argument. It overlooks the existence of the maternal instinct and its possible effects. Perhaps the lady hoped to be allowed to see her children if she behaved to the

L

satisfaction of the Bolshevist authorities. Perhaps, also, she feared that if she did not so behave she might see the inside of one of their prisons for the sixth time.

Directly Mr. Wells arrived in Petersburg he was taken to visit a school. He had a special guide who began to question the children upon the subject of English literature and the writers they liked best. Mr. Wells says, " One name dominated all others. My own. Such comparatively trivial figures as Milton, Dickens, Shakespeare ran about intermittently between the feet of this literary colossus." Mr. Wells concluded that this **was** the result of certain kindly-meant intrigues carried out with the object of making him feel himself at home in Russia. One may suspect from this conclusion that Mr. Wells has had little experience of orientals or of Russians. His modesty makes him underestimate his well-deserved reputation for being clever. His Russian friends certainly knew that he would see through this little farce. They must have carried it out for some ulterior purpose. Probably the idea was to make Mr. Wells feel himself to be their superior in intrigue and thereby to vitiate his judgment in any matters in which intrigue was involved. Mr. Wells's book describing his visit to Russia contains a brilliant description of the ruin produced by communism in practice but the idea seems never to have occurred to him that there is anything abnormal or of psychological interest in the mentality of the Bolshevists.*

---

* *Russia in the Shadows* (Hodder and Stoughton, 1920).

The effect of strange surroundings on mental ability is a matter of serious importance to commercial firms who sometimes have to send young and inexperienced men to represent them in foreign countries. Such representatives are apt to suffer from obtuseness in understanding orders and, in other ways, from a serious lack of judgment. For instance, a young commercial traveller was trying to sell a certain kind of paper at two-pence-halfpenny a pound. It was necessary for him to cut his price. An experienced friend told him that a cut of 1/32 of a penny would be sufficient. He disregarded this advice and reduced his price to 1 7/8d. He sold a good deal of paper at this rate but was dismissed as soon as his firm knew that he was thus selling their goods at a loss. To pick out especially intelligent and receptive young men to be commercial travellers is no remedy for the difficulty but rather the reverse. What is required is that beginners should first spend a year in the country in which they will have to travel in some occupation in which office hours will have to be observed and in which they will be paid a fixed salary and be allowed nothing for expenses.

During my first year in India, when my mental disabilities must have included those of the globe-trotter, it was noticed by me that the Greek alphabet had completely escaped my memory. After a few years, knowledge of it again became available to my consciousness so that it became possible for me to read the words of a Greek quotation and sometimes to recognise their meaning. This return to consciousness was not due to any conscious effort on my part. It is probable that a similar decrease in availability of stored data lies at the bottom of the mental disabilities of the globe-trotter. He feels that he is thinking well and clearly and his opinions seem to him to be logical and above criticism. But his reasoning is concerned solely with the data present under his nose. His power of using past experiences is diminished. It is probable that the stored data that are shut off from consciousness are also shut off from that part of the subconscious mind that has to do with the forming of common-sense decisions. On studying the globe-trotter it is evident that his mental disabilities are not due to fatigue or to ill-heath. The disturbing factor is probably the unusual vividness and interest of his sensory impressions.

Scattered through this book various reasons will be found for believing that data are best available for use in an act of subconscious judgment when they have been forgotten by the conscious mind. Our study of abnormal calculating ability indicated that probably it was not the act of forgetting but the fact that the data were unknown to consciousness that made them thus available. The facts described in the present chapter lead one to suspect that too vivid consciousness is harmful to subconscious judgment because it tends to render stored data less available for use by the subconscious mind.

The foregoing considerations are not meant to suggest that there are no advantages in travelling. A change of scene is a valuable rest for the brain. But it is advisable to remember that when the brain is resting it is not wide awake. Hence if a committee or commission is appointed to go abroad to carry out some investigation, its members would do well to defer writing their report until after their return.

Apart from resting the brain, travelling may do good in widening one's experience of life. An inhabitant of a very small town somewhere in California was once heard to remark, " Paris and London—Yes—very fine cities I presume, but re-mote."

CHAPTER XII

OPPOSITION TO NEW IDEAS

Opposition to railways—Distrust of unknown men—" Alexic "
theories—Hatred—Objection to sensational statements—
Forgetting unwelcome evidence—Tact—Nature of the
critical faculty.

In an earlier chapter of this book a story was related
of the very acute reasoning of Sir Astley Cooper in a
murder case. Anyone reading the story would rightly
conclude that Sir Astley was an exceptionally clever
man. But his reasoning power was not always in such
good working order. He had a strong prejudice against
railways and especially against a proposed railway that
would pass near his property. When George Stephenson, the founder of railways, called on him to try to
persuade him to withdraw his opposition, he expressed
the following opinion :

" Your scheme is preposterous in the extreme. It is
of so extravagant a character as to be positively absurd.
Then look at the recklessness of your proceedings !
You are proposing to cut up our estates in all directions
for the purpose of making an unnecessary road. Do
you think for one moment of the destruction of property
involved in it ? Why, gentlemen, if this sort of thing
be permitted to go on, you will in a very few years
destroy the *noblesse !* "

Perhaps Sir Astley Cooper's opinion on the effect of railways in altering the position of the noblesse was not so very far wrong. But yet his opinion furnishes a good example of prejudice. To say so, however, carries us a very little way towards an explanation. Let us consider some other examples of singularly mistaken estimates about railways. A book entitled *A Practical Treatise on Railways* was published in 1825. Its author was Mr. Nicholas Wood, who, as he was a friend of George Stephenson, might be expected, if he had any prejudice, to have one in favour of railways. His book, however, contained the following statement :

" It is far from my wish to promulgate to the world that the ridiculous expectations, or rather professions, of the enthusiastic speculist will be realised, and that we shall see engines travelling at the rate of twelve, sixteen, eighteen, or twenty miles an hour. Nothing could do more harm towards their general adoption and improvement than the promulgation of such nonsense."

About this time the *Quarterly Review* published an able article on the projected Liverpool and Manchester Railway. As the author was in favour of the scheme, one would expect, if he had any prejudice, that he would form a high estimate of the capabilities of the steam locomotive. But, adverting to another project for a railway to Woolwich, he wrote : " What can be more palpably absurd and ridiculous than the prospect held out of locomotives travelling *twice as fast* as stage coaches! We would as soon expect the people of Woolwich to suffer themselves to be fired off upon one of Congreve's ricochet rockets, as trust themselves to the mercy of a machine going at such a rate."

What is the source of the mistakes made by these two writers ? Had they been asked they probably would have replied that they had heard Stephenson's arguments and had found them unconvincing. Why were these arguments unconvincing ?

We have elsewhere considered instances in which subconscious judgment was superior to conscious reasoning and also other instances in which the unobtrusive help of the subconscious mind was beneficial to such reasoning. Members of a jury would probably assert that they decided by conscious reasoning about the evidence. But we have seen that it is probable that their being convinced by one argument and not by another was due to influences coming from their subconscious minds. Their reason was tempered by common sense. In deciding about affairs of human intercourse, such common sense, based as it is on previous experience of human intercourse, is of value. But such common sense is entirely out of place in deciding about a matter in which previous experience is lacking. Hence common sense based on experience of travelling by stage coaches was of no use in deciding about speeds attainable by locomotive engines.

Such " stage-coach common sense " was probably the source of the following opinion expressed by Dionysius Lardner, at a meeting of the British Association in 1836, in a lecture on steam navigation : " As to the project of establishing a steam intercourse with the United

States . . . it was, he had no hesitation in saying, perfectly chimerical, and they might as well talk of making a voyage from New York or Liverpool to the moon."

Thus one kind of opposition to new ideas has been shown in the past by those who, though relying on reason in dealing with their own discoveries, have left it for common sense when dealing with the discoveries of other people. In recent years new and revolutionary discoveries have followed one another so frequently, especially in the physical sciences, that it is difficult to believe that opposition of this kind will hamper the progress of science in the future.

We have now to consider other ways in which the work of the subconscious mind may be detrimental to our reasoning processes.

We are liable to be influenced by a prejudice when we hear a novel opinion expressed by a man who is not an authority on the subject involved. Instances are known of a man of science being unduly critical when another man trespasses on his preserves. Such distrust no doubt is in accordance with common sense and perhaps more often than not is justified by the event. An instance in which it was not so justified is related by Lord Playfair in his memoirs.* He says:

" Sir Robert Peel offered me an appointment as Chemist to the Geological Survey. . . . Before commencing my new labours, Sir Robert Peel, with that

---

* *Memoirs of Lyon Playfair,* by Wemyss Reid (London, Cassel and Co., 1900).

great kindness which he always showed to me, invited me to meet some of my future chiefs at Drayton Manor. . . . Stephenson, the inventor of the railway system, Follett, the great lawyer . . . were also visitors at Drayton Manor. It used to be Sir Robert Peel's amusement to promote discussion among the philosophers after dinner. Stephenson spoke of locomotives, and how their power was obtained. He offered what was then a daring speculation, that the original source of power in steam-engines was the sun, which conserved its force in plants of which coal is the residue. This is now known to be a truth, but at that time appeared to be inconceivable folly. As the geologists laughed at the theory, Stephenson abandoned the controversy. Next day Sir Robert Peel asked me what I thought of Stephenson's view, because he noticed that I did not take part in the discussion. I told him that the idea was not absurd, and could be supported by good arguments. He then desired me to explain these to Follett, and he would ask him to be Stephenson's advocate at dinner on that day. Follett entered into the spirit of the joke, and readily comprehended the explanations of a possible correlation of forces. Accordingly when the discussion was again raised after dinner, Follett turned the tables on the geologists and completely defeated their arguments. Stephenson looked on in amazement, and exclaimed, " Of all the powers in Nature, the greatest is the gift of the gab ! "

We now come to a source of opposition to new ideas that is of great psychological interest.

It is a singular fact that if one puts forward a suggestion that is objected to, the objection, in nine cases out of ten, in my experience, does not take the form of rebutting evidence : it takes the form of an alternative theory made up on the spur of the moment and that usually will not bear more than a moment's examination. Let us consider some examples.

The explanation of the success of the jury system put forward in an earlier chapter is only one of a large number of proofs contained in this book that forgetting is favourable to or necessary for an act of subconscious judgment. A critic of my former book, to whom I am indebted in other respects, appears to have forgotten each one of these proofs before he came to the next and therefore failed to recognise their cumulative effect. Hence he fell foul of my description of the use of juries. Instead of adducing facts to disprove my view, he put forward a theory of his own, asserting that the jury system is " a direct outcome of an attempt to counteract the want of scientific knowledge of our judges." An equally unsatisfactory theory was put forward by another critic to the effect that the success of the jury system was due to members of the jury being of the same social level as the accused.

In Æsop's fables it is related how a fox having tried to reach some grapes without success comforted himself in his failure by saying that " The grapes are sour." Thus the fox, on the spur of the moment, made up a theory to dispel a disagreeable impression. Let us seek for evidence that other theories made up on the spur of the moment have the function of protecting the mind against unwelcome impressions. Such theories may be termed " alexic " from the word ἀλεξειν, to protect.

For several years past one of my hobbies has been observation of the flight of soaring birds. My only qualification for the task has been a certain amount of industry in observing. My ignorance of ærodynamics and other cognate sciences has led me to make interpretations of the facts which have met with criticism usually if not always well-deserved but yet sometimes containing instructive examples of alexic theories.*

For instance, it has been asserted by me that sea gulls can sometimes remain in effortless gliding flight when in a descending current of air at the stern of a steamer. Two unscientific critics have set themselves to test this assertion. One of them, as the result of observation, asserts that gulls soar near the stern but that no descending current is there present. The other critic finds that there is a descending current at the stern but that gulls carefully avoid it. Each of these criticisms taken by itself is perfectly fair and scientific. But no such fair and satisfactory criticisms have reached me from men of scientific attainments. On telling a very distinguished scientist that gulls soar in the descending current at the stern, he instantly replied, " Then that current must

---

* It has been shown by Sir Gilbert Walker that most of the mistakes in my book *Animal Flight* are due to my having confused ideas on " relative wind." (Proc. Camb. Phil. Soc., Vol. XXI, Pt. IV, p. 363.) Confusion of ideas on this subject is not a matter on which I can lay claim to any monopoly. (*Idem*, Vol. XXII, Pt. II, p. 186.)

have an ascending component." This theory has two characters frequently to be found in alexic theories. First, if it is true, it is nothing more than a statement of fact masquerading as an explanation. Secondly it was put forward without due consideration. With a strange phenomenon the first thing to do is to establish its occurrence : the last thing to do is to explain it. Had my statement related to a commonplace fact, there is no doubt that this scientist, had he criticised it at all, would first have enquired as to the evidence on which my assertion was based. But as it ran counter to the whole of his scientific experience and, if the term is allowed, to his scientific instinct, his subconscious mind instantly presented him with an alexic theory. It attempted thus to repress the disagreeable impression, that some of his fundamental beliefs needed revising.

An interesting example of an alexic theory is the following. An aeronautical authority sent me an account of a peculiar mode of flight of the albatross that had been observed by Mr. Parker Smith. In this form of flight the bird alternately glided with loss of height at low speed and with steep gain of height at apparently high speed. When gliding upwards the bird gained as much height as it had lost when gliding downwards. The successive downward glides were all of approximately the same length. My informant said that the pheno-menon was very interesting, and added, " I cannot conceive of any explanation from any knowledge of aerodynamics which I have at present." But on my pointing out to him a paradoxical consequence of this fŏrm of flight he at once wrote to me in reply suggesting that it may be due to variations in the strength of the wind, the albatross gliding downhill during each lull and uphill during each gust. Thus, at first, my informant could conceive of no possible explanation. But as soon as it had been pointed out to him how greatly the phenomenon ran counter to his aerodynamical knowledge, his subconscious mind immediately furnished him with a theory to explain it. The theory may be true but it deserves the name of alexic as he put it forward without any attempt to enquire whether the gusts were of equal intensity and occurred at equal intervals as must have been the case if they were the source of the phenomenon. His first statement that he could conceive of no explanation suggested that further research was required. His second thoughts, on the contrary, suggested that further research was unnecessary. This is a frequent and regrettable character of alexic theories. Another observer who has seen the Parker Smith form of flight of the albatross informs me that it only occurs in very hot weather. This is the second stage of knowledge of a phenomenon, namely, knowledge of the conditions under which it occurs. It is only after these are known that it will be advisable to begin to seek for an explanation.

Another method by which the mind protects itself from unwelcome impressions appears to be by developing a feeling of hatred. Macaulay, in his essay on Southey's *Colloquies*, says that his author " brings to the task two faculties which were never, we believe, vouchsafed in measure so copious to any human being, the faculty of believing without a reason, and the faculty of hating without a provocation." No doubt to Southey, as to others, evidence that proved him to be wrong was unwelcome and it is probable that he developed a hatred of those who based their beliefs on evidence as a means of distracting his attention from the insecure foundations of his own opinions. Unscientific opposition on the part of men of science to new discoveries has sometimes assumed the form of an irrational hatred. This was shown in an essay in the *Edinburgh Review* on Young's theory that light was due to vibrations of the ether. Till then Sir Isaac Newton's view that light was due to particles shot off from the luminous body had been universally held. The writer says :

" We now dismiss, for the present, the feeble lucubrations of this author, in which we have searched, without success, for some trace of learning, acuteness and ingenuity, that might compensate his evident deficiency in the powers of solid thinking."

The writer's statement that he had done with Young " for the present " appears to be a threat to subject him to further castigation should he venture to again defend his views. The writer goes on to say that he had approached the subject with a mind devoid of any preconceived ideas. This seems to be an instance of " Qui s'excuse s'accuse " for, though our reason may sometimes tell us that we are influenced by a preconceived idea, we have no monitor capable of telling us when we are free of them. A correspondent who once wrote to me on soaring flight with much confidence and little knowledge prefaced his remarks by an identical assertion as to his freedom from preconceived ideas.

The manuscript of the chapter of this book dealing with the mental ability of the Quakers was submitted, by a mutual friend, to an exponent of Quakerism. It was returned to me with such marginal notes as " mere ignorant abuse " or " scarcely rational." The word " preposterous " was written against verbatim quotations from recognised historians of the Quaker sect. Our opinions as to the effect of the mental *régime* of the early Quakers were nearly, if not quite, identical. We differed as to the mode by which this effect had been produced. He gave no reasons, or at least no logical reasons, for his opinions. His opposition appears to have been aroused by the reasons given by me for mine and also to his having very strangely mistaken my writing for an attack on his sect. When my readers come to the chapter in question they will probably be surprised at the idea that it contains anything in the nature of " abuse."

Dr. C. S. Meigs, in a book published in 1852, attacked the idea that certain fevers were due to contagion. " I prefer to attribute them," he wrote, " to accident or Providence, of which I can form a conception rather than to a contagion of which I cannot form any clear idea." He describes the doctrine of contagion as " a vile, demoralising superstition." A clue as to why such opinions were held in face of the evidence that was then already accumulating is given in a speech made at a meeting of doctors held at about that time :

"The result of the whole discussion will, I trust, serve not only to exalt your views of the value and dignity of our profession, but to divest your minds of the overpowering dread that you can ever become the minister of evil ; that you can ever convey, in any possible manner, a horrible virus."

Lord Kelvin, in his later years, appears to have developed a habit of disliking views that were new to him. The following quotation is from the *Life of Lord Raleigh :* "I remember well one visit, probably about 1895, when the now generally accepted theory of electrolytic dissociation, connected with the names of Van't Hoff and Arrhenius, was under discussion. Lord Kelvin had learnt something of it in conversation with friends, and was full of indignation against it. At the same time he showed some desire to learn more of the accursed thing, and a small text-book was produced from Raleigh's shelves in which the theory was expounded. On this occasion he showed more disposition to read than usual, but in a page or two he came across a thermodynamic argument which, if not incorrect, was certainly inconclusive. . . . However, his indignation abated somewhat as he read further." It is further recorded that it was not easy to get him to read half a page of print about anything with which he disagreed. "He would take it up, but the first line or two would send him off on some train of thought of his own, and his eye would wander from the printed page." This appears to be an intrusion of original ideas of alexic origin. Lord Kelvin seems to have had a singular bias against aeronautical matters. He once described Maxim's flying machine as " a sort of child's perambulator magnified eight times." On one occasion he remarked that it would be a long time before men flew about like birds. When, in 1896, he was asked by Colonel Baden Powell to take an interest in aeronautics, he replied :

" I have not the smallest molecule of faith in aerial navigation other than ballooning or of expectation of good results from any of the trials we hear of. So you will understand that I do not care to be a member of the Aeronautical Society."*

Opposition is specially likely to be roused by a discovery that proves not only that an existing belief is wrong but also that the mode of thought that produced that belief is erroneous. For instance, Vesalius is now known as the father of modern anatomy. His great work, *De Humani Corporis Fabrica*, was published in 1543. Its novelty consisted in the fact that he relied on his own observations instead of on authority. His teachings were vigorously opposed. Sylvius, who had been his teacher, declared that the human body had undergone changes in structure since the time of Galen, and, with the object of defending this ancient authority, " he asserted that the straight thigh bones, which, as

---

* When asked his opinion of soaring flight, he replied : " That that puzzled Solomon puzzles me also." It is a plausible guess that this opinion was based on observation of the behaviour of gulls at the stern of a steamer.

everyone saw, were not curved in accordance with the teachings of Galen, were the result of the narrow trousers of his contemporaries, and that they must have been curved in their natural condition when uninterfered with by art."*

Educated people commonly have a prejudice against the sensational. It is possible that this prejudice has sometimes delayed the acceptance of a discovery. Keith says that " our predecessors were largely influenced by prejudice," when referring to their hesitation in accepting the evidence of the antiquity of man. Current belief was then such that any discovery of fossil man would have appeared as highly sensational. Keith's remark referred to such men as Lyell and Huxley among others. Anyone asked to make a list of the most eminent scientific men of the last century would certainly include Lyell the geologist and Huxley the biologist. It is highly improbable that either of these scientists had any conscious bias in favour of the Mosaic cosmogony, but yet, when they came across discoveries that upset prevalent beliefs they were " largely influenced by prejudice." As an example of their scepticism we may refer to the human jaw bone found in the Moulin Quignon gravel pit in north-west France. Huxley was on a committee that examined this specimen and that rejected its authenticity. They concluded that the jaw bone had been placed in the gravel pit by the workmen to deceive Boucher de Perthes, an experienced investigator, who had taken it out of the gravel with his

* Locy, *Biology and its Makers*, p. 35.

own hands. This conclusion appears remarkable in view of the fact that the part of the bone to which the muscles of mastication were attached resembled that of a native Australian in certain striking features and differed in these features from the jaw bone of a Frenchman. It may well be asked where could the workmen have found such a jaw bone if it was really a case of attempted fraud ?

In works on psychology a description may be found of the " defense mechanism " by which the mind seeks to expel or repress unwelcome ideas. That opposition to new discoveries is, in great part, of this nature is proved by the fact that such opposition appears to be mainly at least confined to discoveries that prove that existing beliefs are wrong. A discovery that confirms existing beliefs, or that is merely an addition to existing knowledge, may entirely escape opposition or even receive an apparently undue amount of welcome. As an example it will be of interest to contrast the reception given to the discovery of the planet Neptune and that given to the discovery of the gas argon.

The planet Neptune was found as the result of mathematical calculations carried out independently by two astronomers Adams and Le Verrier. The presence of this planet gave a welcome explanation of certain anomalous movements of the planets Jupiter and Uranus. It furnished a striking proof of the validity of the methods of calculation then relied on by astronomers. But it was not a discovery that opened out new lines of research. It was in a sense the end of a chapter. Shortly

after the discovery had been published, the President
of the Royal Astronomical Society, in his annual address
made a reference to " Le Verrier and Adams—names
which as Genius and Destiny have joined them, I shall
by no means put asunder ; nor will they ever be pronounced apart so long as language shall celebrate the
triumphs of Science in her sublimest walks.   On the
great discovery of Neptune, which may be said to have
surpassed, by intelligible and legitimate means, the
wildest pretensions of *clairvoyance* it would now be
quite superfluous for me to dilate."

The discovery of argon was also one of " the triumphs
of Science in her sublimest walks," but it was a walk
in another direction for it implied that existing beliefs
were wrong.   Its discoverers, Lord Raleigh and Sir
William Ramsay, showed that the atmosphere contained
one per cent. of a constituent whose existence had
never previously been recognised.   When their discovery
was brought before the Royal Society (January, 1895),
a discussion ensued in which " It was agreed by all that
the case for a new gas in the atmosphere had been fully
established.   The admission on the part of the President
of the Chemical Society was, Raleigh thought, somewhat
grudging.   " No doubt the paper will meet with very
considerable criticism throughout the world."   " But
apart from the facts brought forward in this paper, there
is a portion which is purely, one might almost say—if
I may be allowed the expression on such an occasion—
of a wildly speculative character . . . " and so on.   In
fact, Raleigh was somewhat disappointed that dis-

cussion turned almost entirely on the rather dubious conclusion about the monatomic character of the gas as deduced from the ratio of specific heats."* Here we have clear evidence of alexic influences. The above quoted speaker comforted himself by anticipating that others throughout the world would succeed, where he had failed, in making valid criticisms of the asserted discovery. His anticipation can scarcely have been based on any insufficiency of the proof brought forward, for specimens of the gas had been given to other scientists for investigation and their results were published on the same occasion resulting in what was described at the time as " a torrent of new discoveries." It seldom if ever has happened that such complete proof has been brought forward on a single occasion in favour of a new discovery. The discovery of argon was not only a remarkable accomplishment in itself but it was one that opened out new fields of research including the isolation of other gases, such as helium, neon, etc., which were of theoretical and even of practical interest.

An alexic theory may be formed, not only to protect the mind from an impression that suggests that existing beliefs are wrong but also to protect it from incoming impressions that produce a feeling of boredom. For instance, some years ago, when attending a course of instruction in serology, it was noticed by me that my power of assimilating new facts was markedly inferior to that of my colleagues. The subject was one of which

* *Life of Lord Raleigh*, by R. J. Strutt, Fourth Baron Raleigh (London, Edward Arnold & Co., 1924).

I knew little and cared less. My slowness of apprehension appeared to be due to the fact that if any matter was being explained to me, the facts were understood until suddenly an original idea about them came into my consciousness. When this happened comprehension instantly ceased. The original ideas in question were always of an entirely worthless character, perhaps a criticism of the explanation, perhaps an alternative explanation or another way of looking at the matter or even a plan for an experimental test. Many gaps in my knowledge of other branches of science are also due to the obtruding of similarly worthless original ideas. It is especially with subjects that are uninteresting and distasteful to me that such unwelcome ideas appear. A subject that interests me rarely gives rise to an original idea at the time of learning it, but, if at all, usually only on some later occasion when the facts of the case are no longer vividly present to consciousness. It appears that so long as, in popular parlance, one has " an open mind " on the subject, each impression as it arrives is assimilated to its predecessors, but, so soon as the original idea is formed, one no longer has an open mind and then each fresh impression, again in popular parlance, comes in at one ear and goes out at the other. Thus does " the creative faculty of the human mind " assume the character of a mental defect.

Educationalists are aware that it is difficult to make a boy learn well a thing that he already knows badly. The imperfect knowledge of the subject, in some unknown way, checks the entry of better knowledge.

Perhaps it does so somewhat after the fashion of the alexic original ideas just described. Whatever be the exact mechanism involved, the fact of this difficulty appears to be an argument against beginning vocational training at too early an age.

Another method by which the mind protects itself against unwelcome ideas is by forgetting the evidence on which they are based. Darwin, for instance, records that he forgot more easily facts that disagreed with his theories than facts that supported them. If the proof of a new discovery depends on the cumulative effect of a number of petty details of evidence, this alexic forgetting may cause a serious underestimating of its value. One has also a natural unwillingness to recognise the evidential value of facts that tend to disprove one's views. Thus the colleagues of Galileo refused to look through his telescope. It is also difficult to appreciate evidence adduced in favour of a theory with which one disagrees.

Yet another method employed to repel unwelcome ideas is to dwell unduly on side issues. For instance, the *Nineteenth Century* of April, 1877, contains an article by Dr. W. B. Carpenter entitled " A Lesson from the Radiometer." In this it is pointed out that Crookes, when he first constructed this instrument, adopted a mistaken view of the source of the energy that moves its vanes. Similarly it was suggested that Crookes may have been mistaken in his opinion of the cause of the spiritualistic phenomena he was then studying. Carpenter was a biologist and naturally made some mistakes in his description of the radiometer.   A reply by Crookes followed.   It was in true polemical style. It consisted of an elaborate and minute refutation of these mistakes, a matter that had very little bearing on the question whether he was wrong in his estimate of the evidence for spiritualism.

A scientific friend, who was scandalised by my idea that men of science, in common with the rest of humanity, are liable to make alexic theories, suggested to me, as an alternative view, that, in a certain instance, evidence had not been properly appreciated because it had been put before the scientific world in a tactless way.   It is a matter of common knowledge that the chief use of tact is in persuading others to accept one's opinions and no doubt this accomplishment is as desirable for men of science as for others.   Lord Lister's discovery of antiseptic surgery, for example, had as a corollary the imputation that the practice of all other surgeons was wrong.   Unfortunately he brought his discovery to the notice of English surgeons in a way that was likely to hurt their susceptibilities.   At a time when he was a comparatively unknown man, he told his confreres that he could promise them good results if they followed his methods, but that to get the best results it was necessary for them to come to Edinburgh and study under him.   This was scarcely the most tactful way of telling the truth and it is not to be wondered at that surgeons in England were behind continental surgeons in adopting his methods.   But whatever expressions he used, it would hardly have been possible for him to conceal the truth that the success of antiseptic surgery implied a criticism of contemporary practice.

Reasons exist for suspecting that sometimes a line of research is ignored if it promises to upset existing beliefs. One occasionally sees in the newspapers an account of the life of some exceptionally successful man of business who had left school at a very early age or who otherwise had had a bad education. One rarely, if ever, sees similar success recorded of what may be called "schoolmaster's pets." Such evidence that suggests that initiative and ambition may be damaged by too long schooling is commonly overlooked by schoolmasters. They are apt to estimate the success of the education they give by the number of scholarships gained by their pupils at the end of their school career but schoolmasters apparently make no effort to discover what happens to these successful pupils in after life. This appears to be an example of the defense mechanism leading one to ignore lines of research that appear likely to upset existing beliefs. Educationalists, however, are now beginning to realise the necessity for investigating this matter. An educationalist has recently said that education is what is left when one has forgotten all that one learnt at school, an aphorism that suggests that the schoolmaster may be wrong in his persistent efforts to damage that important part of our mental outfit—the mechanism for forgetting.

The facts recorded in this chapter show that the critical faculty is itself not above criticism. Critical power may be an attribute of the greatest minds, but it is a faculty of very lowly origin.   When one is critical one is not necessarily judicial or even logical.   The critical faculty is due to the interplay of a large number of more or less reputable and more or less clearly recognisable emotions that are called into play by what psychologists designate the " defense mechanism."   It may also, in part be due to our reason being unduly influenced by what was described and explained at the beginning of this chapter as " stage-coach common sense."

That we should possess the critical faculty as here described is a fortunate accident, for it results in a demand for those rigorous proofs that are indispensable for the progress of science.

CHAPTER XIII

THE CRITICAL FACULTY OF THE PRACTICAL MAN

*The harmful effects of this faculty—The business man's intoler-
ance of ingenuity—Concealment of ingenuity by Lord
Kelvin—The practical man's resentment at being reasoned
with—Inducing him to use his reason—Unwillingness of
manufacturers to introduce improvements demanded by
their travelling representatvies—The remedy.*

Our study of the critical faculty in the last chapter
has once more exemplified the value of exceptions. The
more or less exceptional instances in which men of
intellect have made mistaken criticisms give us an
insight into the critical faculty of those persons who
may be described as practical rather than intellectual.
With such persons this faculty is often nothing more
than a singular capacity for misrepresenting the evidence
combined with a desire to do so. It frequently causes
them to reject advantageous suggestions. For instance,
at the beginning of the war, it occurred to Sir Alfred
Yarrow, of torpedo-boat fame, that it would be desirable
to start a propaganda in newspapers of neutral countries
to counteract that of the Germans. He made a suggestion to that effect to the Foreign Office without result.
They resented a suggestion made to them by an out-
sider. Sir Alfred Yarrow thereupon began a propaganda at his own expense. The Foreign Office heard
of this ; they requested him to desist and even went to

the length of stopping his letters in the post. It was only at a later date that they were forced to recognise the importance of such propaganda. To take another instance, Lord Kelvin had much difficulty in persuading the Admiralty to take up his different inventions. On one occasion they had received reports from sixty captains of the Royal Navy in whose ships the Kelvin compass had been installed. One report was unfavourable and was made much of. Eight said they had not had sufficient experience. The others were favourable and were suppressed.

It is obvious that if one wishes to influence the judgment of the practical man, it is necessary to let sleeping dogs lie and to avoid awaking his critical faculty. Let us consider, by means of examples, how this may be done.

Many years ago it was related of a prominent member of the Government of India that if he wished to carry any measure, before discussing it with his colleagues, he would contrive to have a short leaderette on the subject inserted in the daily paper that they were in the habit of reading. This they did at breakfast time, when, as their attention was partly occupied with stirring their coffee, the new idea slipped into their minds without the dormant critical faculty being aroused. They were therefore the more ready to agree with it, in that it no longer appeared as a novelty, when it was brought before them at the council table. Naturally the leaderette had to be tactfully written. Had it consisted of violent criticism of government officials for not having carried out the measure, it no doubt would have had an opposite effect.

The value of distracting attention was understood by an officer of the Indian Army who, during a frontier war, was in charge of the intelligence department. When receiving reports from spies he used to have on his table a large bowl full of rupees. The spy, as a reward, was allowed to dip his hand into the bowl and take as many as he could grasp. While telling his tale his eye would keep wandering towards the silver coins and, his attention thus being distracted, he would relate his story without the embroidery with which it would otherwise have been decorated.

It is recorded of the late Sir Andrew Noble, the explosives expert, that on a committee he would often diplomatically ascribe his ideas to some other member. "As you were saying," he would begin his argument. This gentle and unexpected compliment to the intelligence of the person addressed produced a bias and Sir Andrew gained an adherent.

A compliment to be of value must be unexpected and must appear to be accidental. Arthur Roberts, the comedian, once finished a cab drive, somewhere near Piccadilly Circus. As he got out he asked the cabman where he had better go to amuse himself. "Well, sir," said the cabby, "if you want a thoroughly good show and a real good time, you go and see Arthur Roberts at the Pav just over the way there." Owing to this unexpected compliment, Arthur Roberts gave a far more liberal tip than he otherwise would have done.

The cabman was profuse in his thanks but, when driving away, he looked back and called out, in an altered voice, " Good night, Arthur ! "

It is singular how everyone appears to be intolerant of ingenious ideas, or, to be more precise, of the ingenious ideas of other people. One must sympathise with the practical man in his distrust of such ideas. An idea, to appear ingenious, must have about it something unexpected and elaborate. Experience may well show that in the complicated affairs of life such ideas, based as they are on reasoning on a narrow range of data, lead to unexpected and undesirable results. However, this may be in political or social affairs, when we come to deal with the practical applications of science, many of them must necessarily appear ingenious to the uninitiated, but, none the less, are useful in the highest degree. But the man of business is ignorant of this fact. The expert must therefore bear in mind that his ingenuity is likely to be counted against him as a fault and that the more elaborate his reasons the more opposition are they likely to arouse.

Since ingenuity arouses opposition, ingenuity must be concealed. The following is an instance of this being done with successful result.

Lord Kelvin was the author of the plan of furnishing lighthouses with eclipsing lights in order that they could be easily distinguished. The dark intervals in the light were of two kinds, long and short, corresponding to the dots and dashes of the Morse code. A lighthouse might thus flash out the initial letters of its name. Now if

Lord Kelvin had bluntly laid before the Admiralty his suggestion that lighthouses should advertise themselves in this way, the suggestion would probably have been recognised as an " ingenious " idea and as such it would have been opposed and scouted. He, therefore, in the first instance merely suggested that lighthouse lights should have long and short eclipses. Lights so arranged, he said, could easily be distinguished from the mast-head light of a steamer. The authorities consulted used their own reasoning. They realised that they, as practical men, could easily distinguish a light that had a series of long and short eclipses from a light that had none. After the suggestion had been adopted Lord Kelvin allowed it to be known that the eclipses made dots and dashes on the Morse system. In a letter written in 1875 he says : " But I keep in the background the fact that, adhering simply to the letters of the Morse alphabet, we can with the greatest ease give twenty-eight distinctions, each thoroughly unmistakable for any other. This has a tendency to frighten " practical men."*

In the second place, since the practical man's reason is liable to be eclipsed by all kinds of sentiments and prejudices, care must be taken to avoid bringing such influences into play. As an example of an appeal to reason that failed because it also provoked prejudice, an advertisement of a motor bicycle that appeared some years ago may be quoted. " Why be so foolish," it

---

* *Life of Lord Kelvin*, by Silvanus P. Thompson (Macmillan, 1910).

ran, "as to think that because the X.Y.Z. motor-
bicycle wins all the prizes for racing, it cannot also be
used at safe speeds for ordinary purposes?" An
advertisement that began by asserting that prospective
purchasers were fools and that went on to invite them
to consider why they were fools was singularly wanting
in tact and it was not long before the proprietor of the
machine found his way to the bankruptcy court. It is
known to experts in advertising that an advertisement
should never contain a negative. This fact yields a
singular illustration of the insidious effects of suggestion.

It must be borne in mind that the critical faculty of
the practical man is especially liable to be aroused if
he realises that he is being reasoned with. What is
required is to put the data before him with no show of
reasoning on your part and then, if he sees that reasoning
is necessary, he may supply his own. For instance,
Bismarck, in his speech in the Reichstag on the state
purchase of railways, began with a careful avoidance
of any show of ingenious reasoning by comparing the
monopoly that the railways enjoyed to the custom that
had held in France, before the revolution, of farming
out the revenue of the country to certain individuals.
Such a comparison was likely to arouse the reasoning
faculty of his audience and to make them apply it to
the question of the German railways. After making
this comparison, he went on to use reasoned arguments.
For instance, he said that the companies favoured the
foreign producer, who will only bring his goods to them
if favoured, at the expense of the home producer who

must bring his goods to them whether he is favoured or not.*

Another method of gaining assent is the Socratic plan of asking questions. This may be illustrated by the following story :

When Lord Beaconsfield arrived in Berlin for the Congress of the Powers in 1876, it became known to his staff that he intended to open the proceedings by a long speech in French. One of his private secretaries reported this to the British Ambassador, Lord Odo Russell, explaining that unless Lord Beaconsfield could be persuaded to speak in English he would make himself the laughing stock of the Congress. Lord Russell at once went to him to try to persuade him to use English instead of French. " My dear Lord," began Lord Odo, " a dreadful rumour has reached us." " Indeed, pray what is it ? " " We have heard that you intend to open the proceedings to-morrow in French." " Well, Lord Odo, what of that ? " " Why, of course, we all know there is no one in Europe more competent to do so than yourself. But then, after all, to make a French speech is a commonplace accomplishment. There will be at least half a dozen men at the Congress who could do it almost, if not quite, as well as yourself. But, on the other hand, who but you can make an English speech ? All these plenipotentiaries have come from the various courts of Europe expecting the greatest intellectual treat of their lives in hearing English spoken by its greatest

---

* *Modern Germany*, by J. Ellis Barker, 1909, p. 147.

living master.   The question for you, my dear Lord, is,
' Will you disappoint them ? ' " Lord Beaconsfield put
his glass in his eye, fixed his gaze on Lord Odo and then
said, " There is much force in what you say.   I will
consider the point."   And next day he opened the proceedings in English.   Lord Beaconsfield was very well
acquainted with the effect of flattery in vitiating judgment and possibly in this case he saw through it.   But
even if this supposition is correct, Lord Odo Russell's
way of expressing himself is equally an example of the
use of questions in gaining assent.*

The difficulty in using formal reason as a means of
convincing others does not only arise between experts
and practical men.   It also arises in communications
between one business man and another.   This is probably the chief reason for the unwillingness of British
manufacturers to introduce improvements demanded
by their travelling representatives.   The following
incident, told me by an American business man, is an
instance :

A man, who said he was a commercial traveller in
boots, once called at a boot shop somewhere in South
Africa and tried to sell his wares.   The proprietor of the
shop told him it was no use his applying.   He used, he
said, to deal with an English firm.   But this firm
obstinately refused to make boots of the particular
pattern required for use in South Africa.   He had
shown what he wanted to a representative of the firm

* The story is taken from *Collections and Recollections by one
who has kept a diary.*

on several occasions, but with no result. He therefore had to import his boots from Germany. They were not of such good leather as the English boots and did not wear so well. But they had this advantage that they included the little detail that was demanded by his clients. The visitor at length replied that he was one of the partners of the firm in question, that he had heard of the complaints and that he had come to South Africa to see into the matter for himself. Having now been convinced, he consented to make the necessary alteration and was able to renew his trade.

This seems a very expensive way of doing business. The firm first sent out a representative and then refused to be guided by his report. The representative, in writing home to his firm necessarily used logical reasoning. The partners of the firm were accustomed to common sense and could not appreciate such reasoning. It was unfamiliar to them. Perhaps it reminded them vaguely of the sort of " patter " used by promoters of wildcat schemes who attempt to support by reason what is not amenable to common sense. Hence they disregarded the arguments of their representatives. They lost their business and only regained it when one of the partners went to South Africa and learnt at first hand what was wanted.

This firm would have found it a great deal cheaper to have had a representative who could have appealed to their common sense. Let us consider how this could be done.

In the scientific world the value of a man's opinion—

at least if it is a common-place opinion—depends on the evidence he has in favour of it. In government service the value of his opinion depends more on his official position. In the business world it seems to depend more on his salary. Business men, it may be suggested, would do well to pay their travelling representatives such high salaries as would ensure their opinions carrying weight without the help of reasoned argument.

CHAPTER XIV

ON EDUCATIONAL SYSTEMS

Learning modern languages—Mental arithmetic—Classical languages—Scientific education—Education of John Stuart Mill and Herbert Spencer—Methods of developing common sense.

We learnt something about the mode of working of the subconscious mind by studying a naturally occurring abnormality, namely, abnormal calculating power. We may learn something more by studying the artificially produced abnormalities that result from different systems of education.

In describing abnormal calculating ability, we found it convenient to compare the mind to a government office. We shall find that this comparison, despite its vagueness and obvious unreality, will again be of use in classifying the facts that we are about to consider.

Professor Scripture has referred to the ordinary mind-wrecking processes that take place in schools. We may suspect that, in terms of our simile, such ill results are due to some disturbance of the normal relations between the senior clerks, the junior clerks and the director's office.

I. We propose, in a later paragraph, first to consider the effect of learning too many modern languages. So far as the work consists of learning words out of a dictionary, it appears to habituate the mind to learning facts without sufficient associations. In other words, the junior clerks place each impression in a separate file. The results appear to be unsatisfactory except in the case of exceptionally clever persons, who we may imagine to have an unusually large number of junior clerks at their disposal.

II. In old-fashioned Hindu schools in India there exists a system of education consisting entirely of mental arithmetic. We may describe this as a system that involves very little work for the senior clerks and that results in the files being only momentarily considered in the director's office.

III. Old-fashioned education of Indian Mahomedans consists almost entirely in learning by rote a classical language (Arabic) usually without understanding its meaning. In Chinese education also the boys have to spend some years in learning Chinese written characters without understanding them. In both these systems the senior clerks have little else to do than to store the files after their very transient inspection by the head of the office. In Japanese education the children have to learn but also to understand almost the same written characters as the Chinese. In this case the senior clerks have to work and bring their results to the director's office for inspection. Hence Japanese education forms a control for any conclusions we may draw from Indian or Chinese experience.

IV. Such classical languages as Latin and Greek, as they are taught in Europe, because they are highly inflected, result in the pupil having to do a great deal of mental work in recognising the gender, case, tense or number of each of the words. But such work is so uninteresting and trivial that it rapidly passes out of consciousness. It may be regarded as practice in forgetting. In terms of our simile, the files are considered by the senior clerks and brought into the director's office and then immediately sent away.

V. Scientific education, on the contrary, involves constant reasoning and is often highly interesting. In terms of our simile, all the letters brought by the postman are marked "urgent" or "personal." Consequently they are dealt with directly by the head of the office and are not at once sent down to be handled by the senior clerks. We may therefore anticipate that such education, while adding to the power of reasoning about data present in, or readily recalled to, consciousness, must tend to greatly diminish the power to work of the senior clerks. Striking evidence to this effect will be adduced.

I

A story is related of Bismarck to the effect that he was once asked to find a post for a young man who was alleged to be clever because he could speak seven languages. "Then you had better make him into a hotel porter," replied Bismarck, who, presumably, had experience that led him to associate some mental disability with too great a knowledge of modern languages. But it is easy to quote instances of very able men who can converse fluently in two or three languages. Bismarck himself knew five. Two instances are known to me of men of exceptional linguistic ability and clever in other ways who were reputed to be deficient in judgment. The Greek Diamandi, mentioned in an earlier chapter, is stated by Binet to have been aided in his business by his calculating ability. But he had given up his trade when Binet knew him, a fact that gives rise to the suspicion that he had made no brilliant success at it. He is stated to have been proficient in five languages. Similarly in England it is commonly held that foreign correspondence clerks lack the initiative and judgment that would be needed to get them out of their dead-end occupation. Levantines have the reputation of being, as a rule, very clever and astute as business men. But sometimes a Levantine will learn seven or eight languages as well as his mother tongue. Men who have done so are reputed in Egypt to be useless in business. Other evidence comes from Wales where Saer has carried out tests on school children and university students from several districts. He found that those who knew one language only showed considerable superiority in intelligence over those who knew both English and Welsh.*

---

* "The effect of bilingualism on intelligence," by D. S. Saer, *British Journal of Psychology*, 1923, pp. 25-28.

The above evidence indicates that it is not advisable that a boy of average ability who is destined for a business career should, while at school, learn any other modern language than his mother tongue. After his school days are over, he may, possibly with advantage, be sent to a foreign country to pick up something of the language there spoken by practically using it. Words thus learnt as used, with the minimum amount of reference to books, will have other associations than the page of the dictionary on which they occur and consequently we may anticipate that learning them will not stimulate the " parrot memory " in a way that is harmful to the development of common sense and subconscious judgment. Similarly there is no evidence that English children in India incur any harm by picking up eastern languages as they do by conversation with Indian servants. An instance is known to me of a boy of seven years who, having learnt English at home, taught himself five other languages, including Chinese, by talking with shopmen and coolies in the bazaar. He never showed the least tendency to mix up these different languages, owing no doubt to the fact that the words learnt were all strictly associated with the personalities and occupations of the individuals from whom he had learnt them. Hence also languages thus easily learnt by young English children in India are very rapidly forgotten, often apparently within two or three weeks, when they leave India and find themselves in new surroundings.

Lack of knowledge of foreign languages may, no doubt, be an inconvenience to a business man. The evidence we have been discussing shows that an attempt to remedy this inconvenience by teaching a boy foreign languages while at school is likely to have the disadvantage that his capacity for developing the business instinct will be impaired. The late Mr. Pierpont Morgan, the American banker, is reported to have said : " I can hire any expert for 250 dollars and make 250 thousand dollars with the information he gives me. But he can't make the money himself and he can't hire me to do it for him." In the same way it seems that a business man can hire an interpreter while there is room for doubt whether an interpreter can hire a business man.

II

There is nothing in a multiplication table to appeal either to a boy's interest or to his reason. Nevertheless that an education consisting of multiplication tables and little else may aid the development of the business instinct appears to be shown by the following somewhat singular facts.

The Baniya caste is one occupied in trading whose members are widely distributed through a great part of India. In the more old-fashioned village schools attended by boys of this caste, mental arithmetic is the only subject taught. An official report describes it as " a system of mental arithmetic that made the brain reel to contemplate." The first part of this education consists of multiplication tables, some of which are very complicated and which, in some schools, are learnt without the help of books or writing material or even of symbols. The following table will serve as an example :

" Four and a half times one and a half are six and three quarters.

Four and a half times two and a half are eleven and a quarter.

Four and a half times three and a half are fifteen and three quarters.

Four and a half times four and a half are twenty and a quarter.

Four and a half times five and a half are twenty-four and three quarters.

Four and a half times six and a half are twenty-nine and a quarter.

Four and a half times seven and a half are thirty-three and three quarters.

Four and a half times eight and a half are thirty-eight and a quarter.

Four and a half times nine and a half are forty-two

and three quarters.

Four and a half times ten and a half are forty-seven
and a quarter.

After a course of such tables the pupils finish their
education by learning a number of rules for rapid mental
calculations and formulæ for calculating prices. Afterwards, while helping his father in his business, the Baniya
boy may learn sufficient reading and writing to keep
accounts. This education comes to an end at an early
age, usually ten or eleven years.

This education fails to turn out calculating prodigies
but it produces men who are very adept in mental
arithmetic, in money-lending and any kind of trade
needing business instinct. The village Baniya is
generally a grain dealer. He usually keeps his accounts
in his head. At the end of the day he can remember
exactly how much he has sold of each of the half dozen
kinds of grain that he deals in and the total takings.
In towns, Baniyas generally enter such transactions
in account books. Their system of book-keeping is
complicated.

The Baniyas used to be foremost in money-lending
and banking in the bazaar in Calcutta. But some years
ago they began to neglect their ancient system of
education and instead sent their sons to college. The
result has been disastrous to their business capacity.
They are now completely supplanted by the Marwaris,
a caste who avoid western education as they would the
plague. The Marwaris are even averse to sending their
sons to school. They educate them at home and the

chief part of their education is mental arithmetic of the kind above described. It is a remarkable fact that the financial ability of the Marwari community is such that the prices on the stock exchange in Calcutta are governed by Marwari opinion rather than by the opinion of the many English men of business to be found in Calcutta who have all had the benefits of a rational education. As an indication of the wealth of the community the following trivial fact may be quoted. At a particular date some years ago the total number of Rolls-Royce cars in Calcutta was fourteen. Of these no less than ten belonged to members of the Marwari community.

The Marwaris are reputed to keep three sets of accounts, one for themselves, another for their sleeping partner and the third for the tax collector. So far as this reputation is deserved it indicates a serious defect in their system of education.

The business acumen shown by members of the Baniya caste seems to be apparent immediately they leave school. For instance, some years ago an embezzlement case was tried in Agra which was so complicated that the judge and the Indian barristers employed in it had no small difficulty in following the evidence. But some small boys of the Baniya caste, of ten or twelve years of age, were in court following the details of the case with evident interest.

III

In the past Indian Mahomedans have been obliged, on religious grounds, to learn the Koran in Arabic (which is not their mother tongue) before learning anything else. The Koran is learnt, or has been learnt, by rote, without any reference to grammar or syntax and often without any comprehension of its meaning. In addition the pupils learn enough Arabic characters to be able to read the Koran, enough arithmetic to keep their accounts and practically nothing else. As with the Baniyas, the education comes to an end at an early age.

Indian Mahomedans are pre-eminent for their business instinct. In Calcutta and Bombay, the whole of the wholesale trade in certain articles is in the hands of the Mahomedan community. Its members are distinguished for their commercial ability, as shown in trade, rather than by financial ability as is possessed by the Marwaris. The Mahomedans of southern India are known as Moplahs and their predominence in wholesale trade has already been mentioned.

At the present time the learning of Arabic is rapidly going out of fashion, despite the efforts of Government to encourage its study. It is supposed to be so necessary for boys who want to get on in business to know English, that Mahomedans are unwilling to incur the handicap of devoting two or three years of school life to learning Arabic. The Mahomedan merchants of Bombay and

Calcutta, who got their education twenty or thirty years ago, all, no doubt, learnt Arabic. It will be interesting to see whether the next generation of Mahomedan merchants turns out to be as good as the present one in commercial affairs.

Among Asiatic races the Chinese are distinguished for their business instinct and also, as several informants tell me, for another product of their subconscious minds, namely, their sense of humour. Their education resemble that of the Indian Baniyas in certain respects. In both systems, the main part of the education consists in learning by rote things imperfectly understood. In both systems the boys learn their lessons by repeating them aloud over and over again, hundreds of times, while rocking themselves to and fro. In both systems the education comes to an end at an early age. But the two systems of education differ entirely in their subject matter. The chief part of Chinese education consists in learning the names of, and learning to recognise, the written characters of classical Chinese without any understanding of their meaning. The only relief the boy has from this tedious work is that, during part of the day, he is taught to copy the characters on paper. In his second year the boy has to return to the beginning of his primer—the " Three Character Classic " —and commences to learn the meaning of the words that he already knows how to write. Many finish their education at this stage. Others continue it by learning other books in the same way. The second book learnt is merely a list of four hundred and fifty characters employed as family names. All the other books used are ancient classics. After this education Chinese boys learn such arithmetic as is needed for business purposes. This they do easily and well with the help of the abacus. As a proof of their proficiency in arithmetic, it may be mentioned that Japanese banks generally have a Chinese accountant. The reason for this is stated to be, not so much the honesty of such an accountant, as the fact that, owing to the many varieties of dollar current in the Far East, it is only a Chinaman who can cope with the complicated arithmetic involved.

In Japanese education a system of written pictorial characters has also to be learnt. But there is this important difference. The boy learns the meaning of the symbols at the same time as he learns to recognise them. Less time is spent in learning these characters than is the case with Chinese. The Japanese education is varied ; many subjects are taught. It appeals throughout to the intelligence of the pupil.

One system produces men famed for their business instinct. The other system produces men of business distinguished not for their business instinct but for their enterprise and their capacity for taking up new branches of trade.

IV

The next point to consider is the possible educational value of learning highly inflected languages such as Latin or Greek.

Because these languages are highly inflected, the labour involved in learning them is out of all proportion to the knowledge gained. . A boy who has to translate from a classical language has a great deal of difficulty with almost every word. He has to recognise whether it is a verb, an adjective or a substantive. He has to decide whether it is singular or plural, masculine or feminine, or what is its tense or mood. This work may be done subconsciously. If done consciously it is in itself profoundly uninteresting. It makes but little permanent load on the memory. The boy may remember the meaning of the words ; he may remember the grammar, but each individual application of his knowledge is at once forgotten as much as is the labour of turning over the pages of his dictionary. Thus in teaching a boy Latin or Greek he is made to do mental work that he at once forgets. His mechanism for forgetting is thereby stimulated. Returning to our comparison of the mind to a government office, we may say that in such education but little work is done in the director's room ; the files brought there are immediately removed. In this respect classical education resembles education in Arabic of Indian Mahomedans, Chinese education and the education in mental arithmetic of

Indian Baniyas.

The mechanism for forgetting is admitted to be an important part of the mind. It is stimulated by a classical education in the sense that those so educated have the power of passing on data to the subconscious mind and therefore of dealing with them by means of subconscious judgment. In a description of Lord Roberts it is stated that he had the special gift " that, out of the medley of unanswerable reasons, he had an instinct for selecting those which really mattered, and keeping his mind close shut against the rest." What this really means is that he had the power of passing the medley of unanswerable reasons from consciousness to his subconscious mind. The resulting decision arrived at subconsciously returned to consciousness as an instinctive judgment. It was only his conscious mind that was " close shut against the rest." Similarly a newspaper report of Mr. Lloyd George or some other statesman is likely to say that the individual in question has an instinctive power of seizing on the crucial point of any matter with which he has to deal. The implication that his mind works by recognising the important points and overlooking those that are unimportant is no doubt wrong. What happens is that all the different points are dealt with, not by his consciousness, but by his subconscious mind. The resultant of the reasoned decision of his subconscious mind alone returns to consciousness. This mental habit would be fatal to a scientist who must needs have reasons for every stage of the mental processes by which he comes to a decision.   With an affair of test tubes he can only come to a decision when the data available are sufficient for the employment of reason.   With an affair of state, it must often happen that the data available to consciousness are quite insufficient for treatment by conscious reasoning.   On such occasions the statesman must rely on his instinct.   So doing would be impossible if, in terms of our simile, he had the habit of deciding everything by means of the files available in the director's room.

V

We now have to consider evidence of the effects of a scientific education.   In systems of education previously considered the work done has always been uninteresting. Usually it has not involved much effort of conscious reasoning.   In the case of classics conscious reasoning plays a part but the things reasoned about are of such a trivial and uninteresting nature that they would not be likely to occupy the consciousness for long.

Scientific education on the contrary involves much conscious reasoning.   It is often interesting.   In learning a scientific subject, previously known facts must be frequently recalled to consciousness. If a boy learns a number of facts about electricity for example, he cannot understand one without remembering a good many of the others. They are interdependent. A fact of this nature is only learnt when it is understood. Understanding means that the mind brings the fact into relation with previously known facts which, for the purpose, have to be kept within easy reach of consciousness. Thus education in science is pre-eminently calculated to develop the power of conscious reasoning. Let us consider evidence of its effect on the developing mind.

A very distinguished scientist who, some years ago, held a teaching post in an important college was once asked by me whether he was allowing his son to learn science. " Indeed I am not," he replied. " I find that students who come to me who have learnt science at school always do badly at it afterwards. They seem to be bored, *blasé* and indifferent." He told me that, for some reason that he did not understand, the mind of a young boy seemed to be harmed by scientific teaching. On my repeating these remarks to a master at a large school, he told me that it was well-known at his school that if they wanted one of their boys to get an entrance exhibition or scholarship in science at the university, it was of little use to send up one who had had a regular scientific education. He would always be cut out by a boy who had taken classics and who had been crammed in science for three months before the examination. It seems to be a matter of common belief that boys who have learnt science do not do well in it afterwards. The explanation commonly given is that the better class of boys do not take science. It is very difficult to believe such a suggestion. An alternative view is that science boys are not of the better class because of the evil effects of their education. But leaving surmises, let us go on to further evidence.

The following is quoted from Livingstone's *Defence of Classical Education* (Macmillan & Co., 1917) :

" In 1870, as we saw, the (German) universities became partly open to students who did not know Latin or Greek. In 1880, after ten years' trial of the new system, a manifesto was addressed to the Prussian Minister of Education by *all* the members of the Philosophical Faculty of the Berlin University ; it records the opinion of the results of the change which are entertained by the most eminent teachers and savants of Germany. It should be remembered that the Philosophical Faculty in Germany includes mathematics and physical science ; the manifesto was thus signed not only by historians like Mommsen, Droysen and Curtius, philosophers like Zeller, and scholars like Vahlen and Nitsch, but also by the leading men of science in Germany, among them men of world-wide reputation like A. W. Hofmann (chemistry), Helmholz (physics), Kiepert (geography), and by many other scientists. Here are some extracts : " It is also emphasised by the instructors of chemistry that graduates of *Realschulen* (Modern schools) do not stand upon the same level with graduates of *Gymnasia* (classical schools). Professor Hofmann observes that the students from *Realschulen,* in consequence of their being conversant with a large number of facts, outrank, as a rule, those from the *Gymnasia* during the experimental exercises of the first half-year, but that the situation is soon reversed, and, given equal abilities, the latter almost invariably carry off the honours in the end ; that the latter are mentally better trained, and have acquired in a higher degree the ability to understand and solve scientific problems. Professor Hofmann adds . . . that ' Liebig expressed himself at various times to the same effect.' Similar testimony is given by the professors of Mathematics, Zoology, Modern Languages, Economics and Statistics."

It may be noted that the above statements are not evidence that learning science is bad for the adult mind but it is evidence—and very strong evidence—that it is bad for the minds of young children.

The schoolmaster who judges of the progress of his pupils by what they do in the examination at the end of the term is likely to rely on stimulating their interest in their work, interest being a potent aid to memory. The more a boy is interested the more he is likely to remember of his work and the better will he do in the examination. But undue reliance on interest is liable to result in the boy only being able to work hard at a subject that pleases him, whereas in real life he will often have to do with energy things that cannot possibly appeal to his interest. If education is made too interesting then when boys leave school and enter business they are apt to spend too much time in " watching the clock." A report published in 1918 by the London School Committee contains the statement that the elementary schoolboy, after he has left school, is found to be deficient in handwriting, spelling, arithmetic, obedience, thoroughness, common sense and manners. The severer critics on this committee added that the boys were deficient in general accuracy, sense of honour or responsibility, respect to their elders and interest in their work. The public schoolboy was said to be unable to express himself in good English and breaks down at tests of " grit, initiative and ability to grapple with new problems." Thus the effort to constantly arouse interest and stimulate the power of conscious reasoning that one finds in modern education has results that are the reverse of satisfactory.

An experienced schoolmaster informs me that, in his opinion, tit-bits of interesting information are not good for boys. The boy should learn nothing except what he learns thoroughly. An English inspector of schools of my acquaintance even goes so far as to say that he has noticed that boys have less general ability at schools where interesting magazines are taken in than they show at schools where no such attempt is made to stimulate their intelligence. It is probable, in view of what has gone before, that tit-bits of interesting information are bad for boys simply because they are interesting. They remain unduly present to the consciousness and, in terms of our simile, tend to keep too many of the head clerks in the director's office.

Apropos of this subject there is a curious piece of evidence told me by an officer who, during the war, was in charge of a training school for non-commissioned officers in England. " One fact," he writes, " I have established more or less clearly—the effect of close order drill on general obedience. I get six times as many charges (trivial) against N.C.O.'s, now that I try to develop their intelligence, as I did in the old days, when I taught nothing but drill with a view to influence character. Other conditions and type of man practically the same. My experience is based on over a thousand N.C.O.'s."

VI

It will now be of interest to consider two instances in which a hereditary tendency to use reason more than other people was stimulated by an unusually rational education.

John Stuart Mill, the well-known political economist, began to learn Greek and arithmetic when three years old. When taking walks with his father he used to repeat his yesterday's lessons, a practice that must have been a potent aid to memory. He had but few children's books and no holidays. His greatest amusement at all times, he says, was reading about experimental science. Between his eighth and twelfth years he read Virgil, Horace, Phædrus, Livy, Ovid, Sallust and many other Latin authors, besides Aristotle's rhetoric " the first expressly scientific treatise he had read. At the age of 12 he read several Latin treatises on scholastic logic. At 13 years of age he went through a complete course of political economy. He says : " I do not believe that any scientific teaching ever was more thorough, or better fitted for training the faculties, than the mode in which logic and political economy were taught to me by my father. Striving, even in an exaggerated degree, to call forth the activity of my faculties, by making me find out everything for myself, he gave his explanations not before, but after, I had felt the full force of the difficulties ; and not only gave me an accurate knowledge of these two great subjects, as far as they were then understood, but made me a thinker on both. I thought for myself almost from the first, and occasionally thought differently from him, though for a long time only upon minor points, and making his opinion the ultimate standard. At a later period I even occasionally convinced him, and altered his opinion on some point of detail : which I state to his honour, not my own. It at once exemplifies his perfect candour, and the real worth of his method of teaching . . . Mine, however, was not an education of cram. My father never permitted anything which I learnt to degenerate into a mere exercise of memory. . . . Anything which could be found out by thinking I never was told, until I had exhausted my efforts to find it out for myself."

As regards the results of this education, he says he suffered from " general slackness of mind in matters of daily life," and that " the education which my father gave me was in itself much more fitted for training me to *know* than to *do*."

It is of interest to compare John Stuart Mill with Professor Huxley, the biologist. Huxley had a very bad education as judged by ordinary standards. But it included much stern discipline, both as a medical student and afterwards during his four years' cruise on the *Rattlesnake* when he began his important zoological discoveries. He alludes to his life during this cruise as " an education of inestimable value." Previously he had spent two years at " a pandemonium of a school " and, after that, he received " neither help nor sympathy in any intellectual direction " till he reached manhood. Huxley was an able administrator, a man of great common sense, and, in his researches showed, from the beginning of his career, to a remarkable degree, an instinctive power of choosing lines of research leading to important results.

The education of Herbert Spencer, the philosopher, on the other hand, lacked discipline. He began to learn his letters when four years old but, as he exhibited no interest in them, his father ceased to teach him. Hence he was backward as compared with other children He was much left to do as he liked. He was allowed very few nursery books and even these had been expurgated. At a time when other children were hearing fairy stories, his father used to ask him " what is the cause of this ? " or " how do you explain that ? " He used to occupy himself with natural history. He was a frequent listener at discussions on religion, politics and science. He objected to learning the Latin grammar owing to its want of system. He was delighted with trigonometry. He disliked languages owing, he supposes, to his objection to dogmatic statements.

As he grew up he showed but little capacity for dealing with his fellow men. In his biography he mentions and laments two occasions on which he criticised his official superiors, overlooking the fact that each of these incidents was followed by a rise of salary. As a young man he spent much time and energy in matters that a modicum of common sense would have warned him were highly unlikely to lead to useful results in his hands. Though not a chemist, he tried to make crystals by electrolysis, stimulated by " wild hopes of pecuniary success." Though not a physicist, he tried to design a magneto-electric motor. He made a plan for a vast temple though he was not an architect. He studied plans for a universal language, a subject less appropriate for a philosopher than for a naturalised German jealous of the predominence of the English tongue. Though not a printer, he designed a printing press and also a machine for making type by compression for which he tried to raise capital. He lost £150 in patenting a machine for planing wood which led to no practical result. Perhaps his wildest scheme was for a flying machine consisting of a plane, on the top of which the passengers were to be seated, which was to be lifted into the air like a kite and propelled by a rope connecting it to an endless cable. This latter was to extend from the starting point to the destination. It was to be supported on sheaves and kept in motion at high speed by fixed engines. He only discovered that the plan was chimerical when he went into figures about the horse power required.

It was only at the age of 28 that Spencer dropped such attempts to apply his reason to practical affairs and discovered that his peculiar mental temperament fitted him for writing books on philosophy and for nothing else.

VII

Although an educationalist may be expected to see more clearly than the present writer what changes are needed in the present system of education, if the cultivation of common sense is desired, a few discursive remarks dealing partly with the less important aspects of the matter may not be out of place.

In the first place, as an example of a wrong method of arguing, an opinion expressed by the Mogul Emperor Aurungzebe on education may be quoted.

Bernier, in his *Travels in the Mogul Empire*, relates what he calls an uncommonly good story of this emperor. When, after several years' fighting with his brothers, Aurungzebe had at length seated himself firmly on the throne, his old tutor hastened to court hoping to be rewarded for his services. After much delay, he was granted an interview in which the Emperor is stated to have spoken as follows :

" Pray what is your pleasure with the Mulla-ji ? Do you pretend that I ought to exalt you to the first honours of the State ? Let us then examine your title to any mark of distinction. I do not deny you would possess such a title if you had filled my young mind with suitable instruction. Show me a well-educated youth, and I will say that it is doubtful who has the stronger claim on his gratitude, his father or his tutor. But what was the knowledge I derived under your tuition ? . . . Far from having imparted to me a profound and comprehensive knowledge of the history of mankind, scarcely did I learn from you the names of my ancestors, the renowned founders of this empire. You kept me in total ignorance of their lives, of the events which preceded, and the extraordinary talents which enabled them to achieve their extensive conquests. A familiarity with the languages of surrounding nations may be indispensable to a king ; but you would teach me to read and write Arabic ; doubtless conceiving that you placed me under an everlasting obligation for sacrificing so large a portion of time to the study of a language wherein no one can hope to become proficient without ten or twelve years of close application. Forgetting how many important subjects ought to be embraced in the education of a prince, you acted as if it were chiefly necessary that he should possess great skill in grammar, and such knowledge as belongs to a doctor of law ; and thus did you waste the precious hours of my youth in the dry, unprofitable and never-ending task of learning words ! . . . Go ! Withdraw to thy village. Henceforth let no person know either who thou art, or what is become of thee."

Thus Aurungzebe held a belief that is often met with nowadays, namely, that education is merely a matter of pouring a quart measure into a pint pot, that the ingredients only matter and that overlooks the fact that the mind of the student is a pint pot that is strangely modified in the process of filling. Aurungzebe was a man of untiring energy, of extraordinary skill and ability. He suffered from religious intolerance, but otherwise was a man of exceptional capacity, despite the apparent defects of his education.

The case of another emperor, the German Kaiser, may now be quoted. His tutor held the singular belief that a monarch should never be under the influence of any other man. " His ideal of a monarch was one who, while he might perhaps listen to his responsible advisers, would yet stand above them, and pay no heed to them in forming his judgments and making his decisions." A very competent observer, Count Zedlitz-Trutschler, held that this unfortunate belief lay at the bottom of the Kaiser's defects of character. The Emperor, says this observer, had made this conception largely his own. "The consequence was that, thanks to his anxiety lest he should come under the influence of any individual, his inexperience of men and the world left him at the mercy of perpetually varying forces."* The Kaiser's tutor had never understood the saying of Solomon that "As iron sharpeneth iron so a man sharpeneth the countenance of his friend." He was ignorant of the fact that one's character and one's common sense depend on our past experiences and on our having been influenced by our fellow men.

We have further seen that for our past experiences to be at the disposal of our subconscious minds for the purpose of common-sense decisions, it is necessary for them to be forgotten. Hence if education is to aid in developing common sense it must include practice in forgetting. Cramming is generally supposed to be bad because the things learnt are so soon forgotten. An educational authority has recently instanced the cramming needed for the civil service examination as an example of a bad system. He regards it as absurd to choose a man for administrative work in India by his power of scoring marks in an examination for which he has been crammed. But the proof of the pudding does not lie in its ingredients or in how it was cooked. The proof of the pudding is in the eating. Let us consider the results of the system as regards members of the Indian Covenanted Civil Service. The large number of

---

* *Twelve Years at the Imperial German Court* (London, Nesbit and Co., 1924).

subjects in the entrance examination and the high proficiency required in each effectually prevent the candidate from being specially interested in any one of them. Because he is uninterested he rapidly forgets what he learns. Within a few years of his arriving in India he has usually forgotten even the names of the subjects in which he was examined. He has acquired the habit of going through life without any special interests.* He is uninteresting and uninterested. But as one comes to know Indian civilians one discovers that the man who is interested in nothing is a level-headed man who is equally interested in everything. A young Indian civilian, if you ask him, is likely to tell you that his work is monotonous and dull. What he does not tell you and does not seem to realise is that if he is ordered off to an entirely different job at a moment's notice, he will find it equally uninteresting, but he may be relied on to do it equally well. Under the surface young Indian civilians are as much alike as a row of peas in a pod, a proof that their character has been influenced by their education. They don't talk much. They don't write much apart from official reports. Perhaps they don't think much. Their speciality is doing things guided by their common sense. It may be said that they are machines for doing the right thing at the right time. They are efficient and adaptable and usually free of the brilliancy that so often accompanies unreliability. An English professor of chemistry at an Indian

---

* In my experience, if a man has a habit of forming hobbies he is apt to be a failure as an administrative official.

P

university once lamented to me that "these Indian civilians expect us to be able to turn our hands to anything just as they can themselves." The examination that they have to pass before entering the service does not necessarily pick out the best men. Its use is that, being competitive, it makes all the candidates work hard for some years previously, and so lays the foundation for industrious habits. The vocational training of the Indian civilian begins after his administrative work has begun. In his spare time he has to read up Indian law and other subjects connected with administration. At intervals he has to go to Government headquarters to be tested on these subjects by examinations which are not competitive. A rise of salary is granted for each examination passed. Owing to the fact that Indians so often have better memories than Englishmen, it is probable that they will receive less benefit from the cramming system. Hence, as the services in India become Indianised, this system will probably have to be replaced by one based on nomination of candidates.

The facts described in this book give a clue to the value of formal discipline. Its value does not consist in its being dull or exhausting or monotonous. Such accompaniments of formal discipline must be avoided if it is to be used without ill effects. Its use is that it causes the student to do with energy what he does not do with interest. Because the task is uninteresting, its data rapidly pass from consciousness to the subconscious mind. Thereby the mechanism for forgetting is stimulated. The facts learnt and forgotten are probably useless but what is useful is that a habit is formed of rapidly putting data at the disposal of the subconscious mind where they are available for aiding in acts of subconscious judgment. If a pupil sits in an easy chair and reads a novel, no doubt he rapidly forgets the greater part of what he reads. But this is not the form of stimulation of the mechanism for forgetting that is needed. A course of novel reading, while giving unneeded practice in forgetting trivialities, would do nothing in aiding the pupil to put at the disposal of his subconscious mind some important subject that is only learnt with difficulty. This is the reason why formal discipline should aim at making the pupil do with energy what he does not do with interest. If it were interesting it would stick too long in consciousness. It must have a certain amount of difficulty for the reason above given. But harm is done if the lesson exhausts the pupil. What is required is that he should work, and work hard, until he is tired and then at once leave off.

It is tempting to suppose that a broad education is an advantage, not because the pupil will remember it— he will probably forget nearly all of it—but because it gives him practice in tackling a new subject and also may prevent the stultifying effect of prolonged monotony. But there may be certain risks in carrying a broad education too far and especially in beginning it too soon. Macaulay says of a certain philosopher that "he had indeed acquired more learning than his slender faculties had been able to bear. The small intellectual spark which he possessed had been put out by the fuel." We have just seen that the very extended education of John Stuart Mill, on his own confession, rendered him ill-fitted for dealing with the practical affairs of life. If such results are to be avoided, it seems advisable that the first years of the pupil's school life should be entirely devoted to a thorough grounding in the more elementary subjects and that other studies should only be introduced into the curriculum towards the end of his school career. It also appears to be advisable that no attempt should be made, by repeated examinations or otherwise, to keep each subject learnt permanently in the memory; it would seem to be preferable for an old subject to be dropped whenever a new one is introduced. It is possible that, in the future, educationalists will devise some kind of intelligence tests for determining, in individual cases, how far education may be advantageously extended.

The view of the nature of formal discipline here expressed naturally leads to a criticism of the custom prevalent in England of giving children home work to be done in preparation for next day's lessons. An instance is known to me of a schoolmaster who used to give his boarders an extra hour's work in the morning before breakfast and an extra hour at night, in addition to the preparation work done by them in common with the day pupils. He used to be surprised to find that his day pupils were brighter at their work than his boarders. The latter were kept in a constant state of exhaustion by their excessive work. Such treatment of children is nothing less than stupid brutality. Home work has been abolished in Japan with good effect and should probably be abolished elsewhere. Parents would do well to beware of schools whose pupils are exceptionally successful in getting scholarships and exhibitions at the universities. Two instances have been brought to my notice in which such success was purchased at too dear a price. The pupils had been overstrained and were reputed to be fit for nothing in after life. With adults evening mental work often interferes with the night's rest. It is illogical to tolerate for children a practice that is frequently bad for adults.

This book contains evidence that study too long prolonged is as bad for initiative as it is for the development of the business instinct. So many instances are known of men of exceptional ability and initiative who left school at the age of 15 or 16, that it seems inadvisable for schooldays to be prolonged beyond this age. Of the different races in India perhaps the most satisfactory combination of intelligence and capacity in business is shown by the Parsees. Those of them who do well in business commonly leave school at about the age of 15.

What appears to be needed is that a boy should leave school at about the age of 15 or 16, and then at once enter some business where there is scope for his initiative and common sense. A prolonged lazy interval of doing nothing between leaving school and entering business is most inadvisable. When he first enters business his knowledge may not be sufficient for his needs, or it may not be sufficient for some other business that he is looking forward to in the future. If this is the case facilities should be afforded him for getting instruction outside business hours. Evening classes might be used for this purpose. Possible disadvantages in evening work might be avoided if (1) the classes were not continued too late at night and (2) if their subject matter was entirely different from that of the day's occupation. A somewhat different plan is advocated and in use at Antioch College, Yellow Springs, Ohio, U.S.A. The greater number of the students of this college spend part of their time in actual jobs in business firms in neighbouring towns. Each job is held by two pupils who work it in turn for five week spells, each spell of practical work alternating with a spell of education in college. It is hoped that, among other advantages, the practical experience thus gained will aid the development of the intuitive powers of the mind of the student.

Our desire is that education should, if possible, aid the development of the pupil's judgment. We do not mean by this his power of arguing about a few data immediately present to consciousness. We wish him to have the power of calling to mind, for purposes of argument, other data stored in his memory. His reasoning is the better the greater is the range of stored data at his disposal. But for many purposes the best form of reasoning is that in which our opinion is influenced by mental processes and stored data which remain, during the whole process, outside our consciousness. Hence the worst kind of reasoning to demand from the child is that in which hard thought is required about a narrow range of data. The game of chess demands such reasoning and, though it may be regarded as a primitive " war game," it is no good training for a soldier. Napoleon was a bad chess player. Draughts is yet more objectionable. in that it uses a still narrower range of data than chess. Similarly, the mathematical master should be forbidden to set the young child those tiresome and ingenious problems of which he is fond, for instance as to what time after twelve o'clock do the hands of the clock make a right angle with each other and so on. Neither should the master, under the pretence of setting a paper on general knowledge, be allowed to ask such questions as " Where is a robin a thrush ? " and " What duke appears to live on apples ? " Such questions have a close resemblance to those riddles whose answers depend on accidental and silly associations which appeal only to stupid and uneducated people.

The result of our investigation is that there are grounds for believing that attempts to directly stimulate intelligence and to arouse interest, so far as they are successful, may aid the pupil in doing well at his school-leaving examination, but his success will be purchased at the cost of his common sense and capacity for sound judgment in the practical affairs of life. In other words, in education we need more discipline (in the sense in which the word has been used above) and less sense. Before admitting any such conclusion, the educationalist will naturally and properly ask whether any instance can be quoted of such unintelligent education being applied on a large scale and what was its result ? An answer to this question will be attempted in the next chapter.

CHAPTER XV

THE MENTAL ABILITY OF THE QUAKERS

George Fox—Peculiar customs of the Quakers—Education in the Society of Friends—Their beliefs as handicaps to business progress—Decrease in numbers—Histories of Quaker families —Quaker bankers—Quaker business firms—Railways, steam ships and the iron industry chiefly developed by Quakers—Philanthropy of Quakers—Inheritance of their business ability—Quakers as scientists.

If a community adopts a system of education in which efforts to develop intelligence are quite subordinated to the teaching of religious dogma and the use of " formal discipline," and if its members hold a creed in which sensible reasoning about many matters of daily conduct is regarded as a temptation of the Evil One, what effect will such a mental *régime* have on their ability ?   In view of what has gone before, an answer to this question will be of interest.   We shall find it in the history of the Quakers.

This religious sect, properly known as the " Society of Friends," was founded by George Fox in the year 1648.* Besides ordinary theological beliefs that they held in common with other Christian sects, they held certain accessory beliefs, which profoundly influenced their daily life and which were based on reasoning so imperfect and short-sighted as almost to deserve the name of irrational.

* Sewel, *History of the Quakers*, English Edition of 1811, p. 26.

One effect of holding these accessory beliefs was to ensure that none but true converts should join the community ; another effect was to diminish social intercourse between members of the community and unbelievers.   Macaulay* says of George Fox that among his beliefs were " that it was falsehood and adulation to use the second person plural instead of the second person singular.   Another was that to talk of the month of March was to worship the bloodthirsty god Mars, and that to talk of Monday was to pay idolatrous homage to the moon.   To say Good-morning or Good-evening was highly reprehensible; for such phrases evidently imported that God had made bad days and bad nights.   A Christian was bound to face death itself rather than touch his hat to the greatest of mankind.   When Fox was challenged to produce any scriptural authority for this dogma, he cited the passage in which it is written that Shadrach, Meshach, and Abed-nego were thrown into the fiery furnace with their hats on ; and if his own narrative may be trusted, the Chief Justice of England was altogether unable to answer this argument except by crying out, ' Take him away, Gaoler.'   Fox insisted much on the not less weighty argument that the Turks never show their bare heads to their superiors ; and he asked with great animation, whether those that bore the noble name of Christians ought not to surpass the Turks in virtue. Bowing he strictly prohibited, and, indeed, seemed to consider it as the effect of Satanical influence ; for he observed, the woman in the Gospel, while she had a

---

* *History of England*, Chapter XVII.

spirit of infirmity, was bowed together, and ceased to bow as soon as the Divine power had liberated her from the tyranny of the Evil One . . . from these rhetorical expressions [in the Bible] in which the duty of patience under injuries is enjoined he deduced the doctrine that self-defence against pirates and assassins is unlawful."

In their use of the words " thee " and " thou "—the so-called " plain language "—in their habit of designating the days of the week and the months by number, in their refusal to use the ordinary salutations demanded by social custom, in their objection to self-defence, and in their peculiar dress, the Quakers held a set of tenets whose incompatibility with profane reason must have been a matter of daily experience. Those who joined the sect must have been persons whose minds were so constituted that they could easily disregard the results of reasoning that to unbelievers appears sensible and conclusive.*

They also habitually showed an unwillingness to rely on conscious reasoning, which sometimes led to singular consequences. A ship belonging to a Quaker once started on a voyage to America carrying a number of Quaker missionaries. Observations of latitude and longitude would have involved an unwelcome reliance on " profane reason." So, instead of making such observations, they " daily waited on the Lord," and,

---

* The following account of the Quakers is based on information chiefly obtained at the Friends' Reference Library, 136, Bishops-gate, London, whose officials gave me very kind and valuable help. The opinions here expressed are my own. An instance of a singular misunderstanding of the purport of this chapter by a Quaker has been mentioned on page 182 of this book.

with guidance thus obtained, reached their destination after a rather lengthy voyage of two months.

A Quaker assembly once issued orders that fish were not to be caught in their breeding season. Instead of giving a rational sanction for this ordinance, they preferred to give a religious one ; they said that catching fish in the breeding season was in some measure " a violation of the command of God in the beginning, when He blessed them and commanded them to increase and multiply."

Instead of a fixed form of service led by an appointed minister. the Quakers, at their meetings, would sit in solemn silence until one of them, impelled by an impulse from the subconscious mind, would begin a prayer or an extempore sermon. Music was banned both from their religious services and from their schools. They considered that in education it led to " self-gratification and little improvement of the mind."

In meetings for secular affairs they objected to anything so rational as counting votes or a show of hands. Controversial speeches referring to previous speakers were strongly discouraged. One or two members were appointed to act as assessors and come to a decision from the tenour of the speeches.

As to education in the Society of Friends, " a fear that it might interfere with the higher light led, at certain periods, to much opposition towards the higher branches. In 1781, a Friend wrote deprecating any large share of learning for school-children " lest it should be injurious to them, touch their vanity and infect them with the disease of taste and refinement that too much prevails amongst us." In 1705 various " heathenish authors " as Virgil, Horace, Juvenal, etc., were laid aside in favour of the Latin Bible, the *Academia celestis*, and Robert Barclay's *Catechism and Apology*, books which must have been of phenomenal dulness to children. The frame of mind of Quaker school-teachers may be judged from the following anecdote : The Right Hon. W. E. Forster, as a boy at a school at Tottenham, wrote an essay in which he referred to mathematics as the noblest of the sciences. Such praise of a product of pure reason somewhat alarmed the worthy schoolmaster who accordingly wrote on the essay that " all worldly knowledge, even that of ' the grandest and noblest structure ever raised by mental art,' was but dross in comparison with the excellency of the knowledge of Christ Jesus and Him crucified."

According to current views such mental habits and such education ought to be the greatest handicap possible in business affairs. Other handicaps were furnished by certain of their tenets.* In 1693, Quaker overseers inspected shops to see if " needless things were sold," such as " lace and ribbons." " Gilbert Latey, the London Court tailor, lost the greater part of his trade because he could no longer trick out his work with the trimmings that the vain world demanded." Owing to

---

* *The Beginnings of Quakerism*, by W. C. Braithwaite. (London, Macmillan & Co., 1912.)

Religious Societies of the Commonwealth, by R. Barclay. (London : Hodder and Stoughton, 1876.)

their regarding it as wrong to take an oath, even in a law court, it was impossible during many years for them to prosecute anyone by whom they had been defrauded. Their refusal to take off their hats when brought into a court of law involved them in heavy fines and imprisonment.

It frequently happens with religious sects that, when the first fervour has worn off, converts are made who join owing to hope of some worldly advantage. It might be suggested that such success as the Quakers had in business was due to hypocritical or self-seeking adherents of this kind. But such an explanation will not meet the case, owing to the fact that the successors of George Fox introduced a measure that effectually excluded insincere converts. This was the "birthright membership rule" introduced in 1737. In virtue of this rule, the wives and children of Quakers had all the privileges of membership, whether or not they belonged to the sect, including assistance in distress and free education for poor children. Henceforward conversion implied pecuniary liability, while expulsion had the opposite tendency. As a result conversion almost ceased, and there was "wholesale expulsion for trivial causes," especially between the years 1753 and 1820. In 1707, at Aberdeen, a member was expelled for "playing at gowf and other suchlike games." Between 1760 and 1825, "disownment" for "marrying out" was specially frequent. Consequently during this period the number of adherents of the sect rapidly diminished.

Thus during the period of religious depression that

followed the first enthusiasm, the careless and indifferent were being expelled. There was a natural selection in virtue of which those who remained in the community were those who could best tolerate the formalism and peculiar habits inculcated by their creed.

Quakers have never formed more than a small fraction of the population. The only statistics known to me on this point are the following :—

In 1661 the number of Quakers living in Great Britain was 30,000 to 40,000 ; in 1669, 60,000 ; in 1727, 60,000. Between the years 1727 and 1820 there was a rapid decrease in numbers as previously explained.

In 1862 the number of Quakers living in Great Britain was 17,034 ; in 1876, under 17,000 ; in 1920 it was 19,130.

After this brief review of the history of the Quakers we may proceed to consider what success they had in business.

In the first place it must be recognised that their honesty gave them an advantage in trading. Until the time of the Quakers, anyone going into a shop in England had to haggle and bargain about the price or stand a risk of being cheated. The Quakers held it dishonest to ask one price and to accept another. Hence they introduced fixed prices, a custom that gave them a substantial advantage early in the history of the movement. George Fox, referring to the confidence in Quaker tradesman thus produced, says in his journal, " and yt last they might send any childe and bee as well used as ymselves att any of there shoppes."

But honest men have failed in business before now. For success the business instinct is indispensable. This the Quakers showed to a remarkable extent. This capacity they exhibited from the first, at a time when they were being subjected to severe persecution. Indeed, whenever the history of Quaker families is sufficiently known it appears that success in business often began at the time of or shortly after their conversion. It will be of interest to quote some examples.

A well-known Quaker family is that of the Gurneys. They are descended from Hugh de Gournay who came over to England with William the Conqueror. Manors and lands were given to the family in Norfolk and Suffolk. They owned a vast territory in Normandy, which was lost to them in 1204. A descendant, Anthony Gurnay, married an heiress in the reign of Henry VIII, but his estate was much diminished during his life time by the sale of several manors. Henry Gurnay, of West Barsham, who died in 1623, in his will bequeathed the reversion of £200 to his younger sons " so that none hould any fantastical or erronious opinions as adjudged by our Bishop or civill lawes." The beginning of interest in religious matters, thus indicated, was not accompanied by any success in business. It is recorded that the later generations of the family at West Barsham were in straitened circumstances. One of the sons of Henry Gurnay was a clergyman. Another, Francis, wsa a merchant who became bankrupt. The grandson of Francis, John Gurnay (later spelt Gurney), born in

1655, became a Quaker and was the founder of the wealth of the Gurney family. He was a silk merchant in Norwich. A descendant of his, Hudson Gurney, F.R.S., wrote in his diary in 1850 :

> " John Gurney, 1670, was a thriving merchant of
> Norwich, worth £20,000,
>
> John Gurney, his grandson, died 1770, worth
> £100,000,
>
> and I, the grandson of the last, wind up 1850,
> worth £800,000."

The banking firm of John and Henry Gurney & Co. was founded in 1775. In 1838 this bank was described as of a power inferior to no banking establishment in Great Britain, that of the Bank of England alone excepted. It is of interest to notice that Hudson Gurney was disowned by the Friends in 1804 for sending a subscription to a fund for volunteers.

Lest it should be thought that a Quaker becoming a banker was an exceptional occurrence, it may be stated here that the number of English country banks founded by Quakers was far out of proportion to the numbers of this small community. English banking originated from some Italian merchants whose business it was to transmit to Italy the revenues drawn from England by the Pope. Lombard Street in London was named after them in 1318, but banking properly so-called only began to develop there about the year 1685. But it is mainly to the Quakers that belongs the credit of having founded a system of banks in country towns in England that for long was " the wonder and admiration of Europe."

To return to our consideration of Quaker families, we may next mention the Barclays of Ury in Scotland. They are descended from Theobald de Berkeley, who was living about 1140. One of his descendants, David Barclay, born in 1580, is recorded as having sold estates that had been in the possession of the family for 530 years. A later descendant was Robert Barclay " the Apologist" (1648-1690), one of the earliest of the Quakers. His controversial writings prove that his capacity for conscious reasoning was well-developed. He showed no capacity in business, but his son was a successful London merchant. He had four grandsons, of whom three became bankers. Their descendants founded the important London bank till lately known as Barclay, Bevan, Tritton & Co.

As regards the Hoare family of bankers, it is known that a Major Hoare went from Devonshire to Ireland as an officer of Cromwell's army. He had five sons. Four of these did not become Quakers and no records are known as to their having shown business capacity. The remaining son, Francis, joined the Society of Friends, and afterwards was a merchant and a banker in Cork. Francis had a son, Samuel, who was a London merchant in the provision trade. The son of Samuel, also named Samuel (1751-1825), was a banker in London and founded the present firm. The first Samuel came to London carrying nothing but a wallet on his back. This is the origin of a wallet carved in stone to be seen

Q

at the present day over the door of Hoare's Bank in Fleet Street.

Quakers early obtained a reputation for shrewdness in business affairs. This shrewdness may be illustrated by the following story of Jonathan Backhouse, a Quaker banker.

A commercial traveller, staying at an inn, and being somewhat elevated after his dinner, began to boast of his wealth, and also to ridicule a stranger who was present dressed in the sombre garments then affected by the Friends. Pulling out a bundle of currency notes he offered to bet that no one present had so much money. The stranger refused to bet but offered to burn a note if the traveller would do likewise. Suiting the action to the word, the Quaker produced a note and lit it in the candle. The commercial traveller imitated him. The Quaker then suggested burning another. The traveller refused, being somewhat sobered by the prospect of losing more. " I am sorry for that," replied the Quaker, " for the note you burnt was on my bank and had you presented it I should have had to pay you five pounds. The one I burnt merely cost me the paper it was printed on."

Tangye's pumps and engines are known all over the world. The founder of the firm, Sir Richard Tangye, a Quaker, was a grandson of an agricultural labourer of the Methodist persuasion. Richard's father, a miner, joined the Wesleyans and afterwards became a Quaker. The grandfather was extremely religious. As a boy, Richard was made to read hymns on Sunday afternoons to his grandfather who invariably preferred the most depressing of Wesley's hymns and was particularly fond of those used at funerals. Thus in this case also the first appearance of religious fervour was not followed by the power of making money. This power only appeared after the family had joined the Quakers. Sir Richard Tangye had singular energy and initiative. It is recorded of him that " His judgment, . . . was a valuable asset to the firm. He had a remarkable power of coming to a quick decision on any matter of business however complicated, which was put before him. He would listen attentively to all that was said, and then saying " Stop a minute " would take a few quick nervous strides up and down the room and come to a decision which he had the faculty of expressing in pithy incisive terms. . . . " There is only one course to pursue " was his method of beginning when he had mastered the facts, and the method which he suggested, in nine cases out of ten, proved to be correct. He would himself have been at a loss, not infrequently, to explain the process by which he arrived at his decision."

It has been suggested that the success of Quakers in business was due to habits of quiet meditation produced by their religious belief. Quiet meditation is slow conscious reasoning. The above description of Sir Richard Tangye's methods show that his success was not due to slow reasoning but to rapid subconscious decision. His power seems to be similar to that of doctors who can make a rapid diagnosis without being able to give reasons for it.

Richard Hanbury (1647-1714) was one of the earliest members of the Society of Friends. He had inherited lands and was engaged in business. His grandson John was known throughout Europe as " the greatest tobacco merchant of his day, perhaps in the world." The grandson of the last was the first Hanbury of the Quaker firm of Truman, Hanbury & Co., brewers.

At one time almost every town in England had a Quaker wine merchant, or a Quaker brewer, or a Quaker maltster. Among Quaker breweries are, or rather were, Walkers, Parkinson, Allens, Hanbury, Barclay and Perkins. Owing to the temperance movement, in which Friends played an important part, Quakers have now given up the trade in alcoholic beverages.

More often the evidence available as to the origin of the business ability of Quakers is less complete than in the above instances. Available records show that many large business firms were founded by them, and there is no evidence that their non-Quaker ancestors had any conspicuous success in commerce.

The shrewdness of Quakers in business matters is shown in their preference for businesses that supplied articles or conveniences for which there was a great public demand.

John Horniman, a Quaker, a self-made man, born in 1803, was a retailer of tea by which he made a fortune and died worth more than £300,000.

Zephaniah Fry, born in 1658, was a follower of George Fox. His grandson, Dr. Joseph Fry, purchased a

patent for making cocoa and founded the firm of S. F.
Fry and Sons, cocoa manufacturers of Bristol. Francis
(1803-1886), the grandson of Dr. Joseph Fry, greatly
enlarged the firm. He was a pioneer of railway enterprise and played an active part in the agitation for
abolition of the slave trade.

Rowntree & Co., of York, is another well-known cocoa
manufacturing firm of Quaker origin.

The firm of Cadbury, cocoa manufacturers of Birmingham, was founded by a Quaker of whom it is recorded
that a piano was never allowed in his house, and who
never sat in an easy chair till he reached the age of 60.
He had twelve employees when he gave over the business
to his two sons. Under their hands it grew till it
employed 3,400 workmen.

Quakers early recognised the wide demand for
medicines. Names of well-known firms of chemists and
druggists of Quaker origin are shown in the following
list :—

	Date of founding or (in brackets) dates of life of founder.
Allen and Hanbury ..	.. (Allen, 1770-1843).
Corbyn	.. (T. Corbyn, 1711-1791).
T. Bell and Sons ..	.. (J. Bell, 1774-1849).
Howards	.. 1793.
Reynolds and Bransome	.. 1816.

The son of J. Bell was the founder of the Pharma-
ceutical Society.

Perhaps the most remarkable example of the foresight
and shrewdness of the Quakers is the part they played

in the introduction of railways and steam navigation. Friend Edward Pease (1767-1859) aided George Stephenson in his experiments. It is recorded that he watched Stephenson running alongside his first locomotive stoking its furnace. At this time mechanical transport was unknown but yet the sight of this imperfect machine encouraged Pease and other Quakers to furnish capital for the first railway ever made, namely, the Stockton and Darlington line (1821). This was long known as the "Quaker Line." Pease also provided part of the capital for the first factory for steam locomotives. Other Friends were the backbone of the Liverpool and Manchester line. Friend Francis Fry, the cocoa manufacturer, has already been mentioned as a pioneer of railway enterprise. Friend John Ellis (1789-1862) promoted the Leicester and Swannington Railway and was the originator of the Midland Railway, of which his son, E. S. Ellis (1817-1879), was afterwards chairman. William Hutchinson was another Quaker manager of the same railway. "In the matter of rails Friend Ransome devised the best form of chair for holding them." His father invented chilled iron plough shares and founded a large business in agricultural implements at Ipswich. Charles May devised the compressed oak trenails for pinning the rails to the ties. "When the lines began working under a cumbrous system of passenger booking, continued from the coaching days, it was Friend Edmundson who devised the present effective system of railway tickets, and likewise invented the machine in general use for stamping them, and it is

Friend Bradshaw who still enlightens the public as to train movements by his Time Tables."*

Quakers were also prominently connected with early steam navigation. Sir Samuel Cunard (1787-1865) was of Quaker descent. Friend James Beale (c. 1798-1879) sent the first steamer across the Atlantic. This was the Sirius, which started on its voyage on March 31st, 1838.

Friend Joseph Robinson Pim (1787-1858) founded the St. George Steam Packet Co., running between England and Ireland, in 1824. He was described in 1835 as " an Irish Friend well known as principal manager of, I suppose, nearly half the steam packets in the kingdom."†

This work of the Friends in introducing mechanical transport was made possible largely through the enterprise of other Quakers. For instance, Matthew Boulton, went into partnership with Watt and enabled the steam engine of the latter to become a commercial success.

The English iron industry perhaps would have dwindled to nothing, owing to exhaustion of supplies of charcoal used in smelting, had it not been for the discoveries of the Quaker ironmaster Abraham Darby, who, perhaps with the assistance of some workmen brought by him from Holland in 1704, at length discovered how

---

* *The Friends : Who they are and what they have done*, by William Beck. (London : Edward Hicks, 1893.)

† " Irish Friends and Steam Navigation," *Journal of the Friends' Historical Society*, Vol. XVII, No. 4, 1920, p. 105. This is based on an article in the *Journal of the Cork Historical and Archæological Society*, 1917, Vol. XXIII.

to use coke in blast furnaces. In 1708 he acquired iron-works at Coalbrookdale and, in the following year, first produced coke-smelted iron on a commercial scale.

According to Ashton, " the more important chapters in the history of the iron industry might be written almost without passing beyond the bounds of the Society of Friends. At one time or other Quakers were to be found conducting ironworks in each of the chief centres of production."*

Bryant and May, who founded the well-known match making business in about 1840, were both Quakers. Among other Quaker firms may be mentioned Huntley and Palmers, biscuits, founded in 1841 ; Reckitt and Sons, blue and starch (1840-1850) ; Thomas Hoyle and Sons, dyers, before 1788 ; R. and J. Beck, opticians (R. Beck, born 1827) ; Hoyle, calicoes ; Christy, hats (1777-1846) ; Ashworth's, cotton manufacturers (H, Ashworth, 1794-1880) ; Were and Fox, woollens (1768) ; Bright and Co., cotton spinning, 1809 (later the Right Hon. John Bright was the head of the firm) ; Joseph Fry, banker and tea shipper (1777-1861) ; Jeremiah Head, banker in Ipswich ; William Cookworthy was the first discoverer of English china clay and founded a por-celain manufacture about 1745.

Among distinguished men of Quaker ancestry may be mentioned : Sir Walter Scott, novelist ; Lord Macaulay, historian ; Sir H. Rawlinson, expert in cuneiform in-scriptions ; Lord Lyndhurst ; Sir Jonathan Hutchinson,

---

* *Iron and Steel in the Industrial Revolution*, by T. S. Ashton. (Manchester University Press, 1924.)

surgeon ; Dr. Tregelles, Biblical scholar ; Abraham Lincoln ; Lindley Murray, author of an English grammar that went through 200 editions ; Thomas Rickman, architect ; Benjamin West, artist and president of the Royal Academy ; the Right Hon. James Wilson, founder of the *Economist* ; Hoover, the American statesman.

At this point in the history of the Quakers it will be well to pause and see whether any conclusion can be drawn from the above-related remarkable facts.

It is fully demonstrated by the above account that the Quakers had exceptional business ability. As to the cause of this ability, it might be suggested that it was due to their religious creed, which might aid in making them honest, or in preventing them from wasting their money in dissipation, or that it gave them habits of calm meditation, or that it made them industrious or thrifty, or that it made them ready to give each other assistance. All these more or less plausible suggestions appear to be, in great part, excluded by the history of another religious sect, namely, that of the Mennonites.

This sect whose creed was formulated in 1632 had theological beliefs that were almost identical with those of the Quakers. They resembled the Quakers also in their endogenous marriage customs, in their objection to military service and war, in their having been subjected to persecution, in their moral and puritanical habits and in being restricted in numbers. They have spread chiefly in America, Holland, Germany and Russia. In matters of belief and custom they differed from the Quakers solely, so far as available information goes, in lacking most if not all of the accessory quasi-rational beliefs that distinguished the Society of Friends. Further research on this point is, however, needed Though members of this sect are known as honest men and as industrious workers, no reason could be found, in books about them studied by me, for ascribing to them any special mental ability in business or otherwise.

That no purely religious influence was the source of the business instinct of the Quakers is also made probable by the fact that they showed high business ability during what a Quaker authority describes as " the darkest period in the history of this church " (c. 1727-1820), when their quasi-rational customs formed perhaps the predominating part of their creed, and that when this dark period was brought to an end by a religious revival and the Quakers gradually dropped their peculiar social customs, their ability (as regards originating apart from maintaining businesses) certainly did not increase and may have diminished.

A further proof that religion was not directly the source of their business ability is that their religion gave them, in a pre-eminent degree, charity—that greatest but least logical of the virtues. Their business instinct enabled them to make money. Their religion impelled them to give it away. Quakers originated most of the philanthropic movements of the nineteenth century.

The British pride themselves on the abolition of slavery. But the first protest against slaveholding came in the year 1688 from German Quakers settled in the United States. The movement soon spread among the Friends.

They refused to own slaves in 1758. The first petition to Parliament on the subject of slavery was presented by Quakers in 1783. When the Society for the Abolition of the Slave Trade was founded in 1787, the great majority of its members were Friends. The movement was carried to success, after years of strenuous agitation, in 1833.

A Quaker, Dr. Thomas Hodgkin (1798-1866), founded the Aborigines Protection Society.

A Quaker, Samuel Bowlby (1802-1884), was an advocate of temperance reform.

Elizabeth Fry and Stephen Grellet, both Quakers, continued John Howard's work of prison reform in 1813. On her first visit to Newgate, Elizabeth Fry discovered that no clothes were provided for children born there. On leaving the prison, filled with generous indignation, she went to a shop, bought flannel, needles and cotton and then sent messages to her friends inviting them to come to her house that same afternoon. This they did and began at once, with their own hands, to make the much-needed garments for the little ones.

William Allen (1770-1843) and Joseph Lancaster (1798-1838), both Quakers, were active workers for the extension of education. Quakers also were responsible for amelioration in the punishment inflicted in schools. At Ackworth, a Quaker school, punishments were only allowed to be settled at weekly courts and it was laid down that whipping should not be inflicted by a master who had been offended, but by another.

Quakers played a prominent part in the agitation for

the abolition of capital punishment for trivial crimes. As a result of this agitation the death penalty was abolished in the case of one hundred and sixty offences.

Peter Bedford, a Quaker (1780-1846), originated soup kitchens, clothing clubs and other means for aiding the poor.

Humane methods of treating lunatics were introduced by William Tuke (1732-1822), Lindley Murray (1745-1826) and other members of the Society of Friends. As a result of this, a general adoption of humane methods occurred at the passing of the Lunacy Act some fifty years later. The York Retreat, an institution for the insane, was founded by Quakers in 1792.

Dr. Dimsdale, F.R.S., a Quaker (1712-1800), played a prominent part in popularising inoculation for small-pox.

Another instance of a combination of religious fervour with business ability is offered by the Moplahs of southern India mentioned in an earlier chapter. Their religion has, as a bye-product, not charity but intolerance under the influence of which they occasionally indulge in terrible orgies of loot and murder of their Hindu neighbours.*

Thus the evidence indicates that, in the case of the Quakers, we must seek the source of their business ability, not in religion or in any virtues fostered by it, but in the influence of education and quasi-rational

---

* In the *Koran* there is " a perpetual inculcation of mercy, almsgiving, justice, fasting, pilgrimage and other good works " (Draper), showing that extreme and cruel intolerance is by no means a necessary part of the Mahomedan religion.

beliefs on their mentality. This influence, aided by
their fear of "self gratification," led them to avoid
filling their memories with interesting data. Consequently their reasoning processes tended to involve
more work of the subconscious mind than would have
been the case had their memory been stimulated by the
learning of interesting subjects. If a Quaker had to
decide any important matter, instead of reasoning about
it, he would pray and wait for an impulse from the subconscious mind. Thus he had practice in arriving at
intuitive decisions as a religious duty. Even Quaker
children, both in England and in America, had practice
in arriving at rapid unreasoned decisions owing to the
fact that they were taught that changing their minds
was equivalent to telling a lie. If a child asked for cake
he had to have it. He was not allowed to change his
mind and ask for jam, and whatever he took he was
obliged to eat.

An affinity between business enterprise and religious
nonconformity has been noticed by several writers.*
It might be suggested that the spirit of enterprise that
led to nonconformity was the cause rather than the effect
of success in business. But the Moplahs in southern
India show business ability combined with religious
fanaticism which is completely orthodox. The early
Mahomedans had a quality allied to business instinct,
namely, administrative ability, which was shown by
them in founding an empire reaching from Bagdad to
Spain. Probably their conversion to this religion was

---

* Ashton, *loc. cit.*, p. 211.

more due to fear of having their heads cut off or to credulity than to what is properly called enterprise.

Converts to Mahomedanism, before their conversion, no doubt, like other uncultivated races, held that all accidents, famines, illnesses or other misfortunes, were due to the activity of evil spirits. From their daily experience they no doubt could quote what they regarded as convincing proofs of such influence. No other explanation of illness or accident was known to them. The founder of Mahomedanism demanded from his followers that they should discard all such results of sensible reasoning. Hence, however rational Mahomenanism may appear to us, however rational it may have appeared to later generations of the followers of Islam, at its inception it was a religion that, like Quakerism, discouraged reliance on profane reason.

We have now to consider some remarkable facts, which, though unanticipated and though they show us that we yet have much more to learn, do not disprove the suggested relation between the mentality of the Quakers and their business ability.

In the first place this ability seems often to have become hereditary. Histories of Quaker families show that business ability has often appeared in several successive generations. In some of the instances quoted, a son or a grandson has shown greater ability than that possessed by the founder of the firm.*

---

* Ashton (*loc. cit.*, p. 216), gives a genealogical table of the Darby family showing business capacity of numerous members in seven generations.

Two possibilities suggest themselves. Either this is a true instance of inheritance of an acquired character or the result was due simply to like influences producing like results in a series of generations. That the former alternative represents the truth is made probable by the fact that, as happens with non-Quaker families in which business ability is inherited (*e.g.*, the Rothschilds and the Barings), in later generations individuals occasionally appear having literary or scientific aptitude in addition to or in place of business ability. Such scientific ability of Quakers is not merely due to a young man preferring to catch butterflies to working in an office. It has often been of an exceptional character and combined with great industry. A Quaker scientist of my acquaintance, who worked with exceptional industry at the university, now writes to me complaining of his " total lack of business instinct and incapacity for quick decision."

One would not anticipate that a small community of religious fanatics should be an important recruiting ground for the Royal Society of London. But this in fact is what has happened.

Quakers who have had the distinction of being elected F.R.S. include Thomas Young (1773-1829), the originator of the undulatory theory of light ; Luke Howard (1772-1864), a pioneer in meteorology ; John Dalton (1766-1844), who first made an estimate of the relative weights of the atoms and thereby placed the atomic theory on a secure basis ; Joseph Jackson Lister (1786-1869), who made important improvements in achromatic lenses ; his son, Lord Lister (1827-1912), the discoverer

of antiseptic surgery ; and Silvanus Thompson (1851-
1916), the electrician. The following is a list of Fellows
of the Royal Society who are Quakers or of Quaker
descent. It fails to show the full influence of Quaker
blood on the Society. For instance, it does not include
Sir Francis Galton whose father was a Quaker. who
" married out " to the daughter of Dr. Erasmus Darwin.

LIST OF FELLOWS OF THE ROYAL SOCIETY OF LONDON
WHO ARE QUAKERS OR OF QUAKER DESCENT FROM
DATE OF FOUNDING OF THE SOCIETY UP TO THE
YEAR 1915 :—

Name.	Born.	Died.	Elected.
Sir John Finch	1626	1682	1663
Anthony Lowther..	—	1672	1663
Richard Lower, M.D.	1631	1691	1667
William Penn	—	—	1681

TOTAL, 1663-1700 : 4.

	Born.	Died.	Elected.
Richard Mead, M.D. (author of books on the plague and on poisons)	1673	754	1703
Fettyplace Bellers (lawyer) ..	—	—	1711
John Bellers (social reformer) ..	1654	1724	1718
George Graham (clockmaker, writer on magnetism and astronomy)	—	1751	1720
Silvanus Bevan	—	—	1725
Peter Collinson (botanist) ..	1693	1768	1728
Thomas Birch, D.D. (historian ; parents Friends)	1705	1766	1734
Richard Brocklesby, M.D. ..	1722	1797	1746

TOTAL, 1701-1750 : 8.

LIST OF FELLOWS OF THE ROYAL SOCIETY—*(continued)*.

Name.	Born.	Died.	Elected.
John Fothergill, M.D. (founder of Ackworth School)	1712	1780	1763
Thomas Dimsdale, M.D. (popularised inoculation for smallpox)	1712	1800	1769
John Coakley Lettson, M.D. (naturalist)	1744	1815	1773
Samuel Galton (great-grandfather of Sir Francis Galton)	1720	1799	1785
Jeremiah Dixon (astronomer) ..	1733	1778	1790
Mark Beaufoy	1764	1827	1790
Thomas Young, M.D. (originator of undulatory theory of light) and Egyptologist	1773	1829	1794

TOTAL, 1751-1800 : 7.

	Born.	Died.	Elected.
Lewis Weston Dilwyn (parents Friends, M.P. for Glamorganshire)	1778	1855	1804
William Allen (chemist and philanthropist)	1770	1843	1807
Robert Willan, M.D.	1757	1812	1809
John Sims	1749	1831	1814
Michael Bland	—	1851	1816
Hudson Gurney	1775	1864	1818
Luke Howard (a pioneer in meteorology)	1772	1864	1821
John Dalton (author of the theory of proportional atomic weights)	1766	1844	1822

R

LIST OF FELLOWS OF THE ROYAL SOCIETY—*(continued)*.

Name.	Born.	Died.	Elected.
John Scandrett Harford (left Friends)	1785	1866	1823
Richard Phillips (chemist) ..	—	—	1827
James Cowles Pritchard, M.D. (author of *Natural History of Man*, etc. ; left Friends) ..	1786	1848	1827
William Phillips (mineralogist and geologist)..	1775	1828	1827
Joseph Jackson Lister (investigator of achromatic lenses)	1786	1869	1832
William Allen Miller	1817	1870	1845
William West	—	—	1846
Robert Were Fox (magnetism and geology)	1798	1877	1848
John Fletcher Miller (meteorologist and astronomer)	1816	1856	1850

TOTAL, 1801-1850 : 17.

	Born.	Died.	Elected.
Charles May	—	—	1854
Isaac Fletcher (left Friends) ..	—	—	1855
Joseph Lister, afterwards Lord Lister (discoverer of antiseptic surgery ; left Friends)	1827	1912	1860
Daniel Oliver (keeper of herbarium at Kew)	—	—	1863
William Pengelley (geologist) ..	1812	1894	1863
Daniel Hanbury (chemist ; parents Friends)	1825	1875	1867

LIST OF FELLOWS OF THE ROYAL SOCIETY—*(continued)*.

Name.	Born.	Died.	Elected.
Edward Burnett Tylor (anthropologist ; left Friends)	—	—	1871
Wilson Fox, M.D. (of Quaker descent)	1831	1887	1872
John Eliot Howard (chemistry of quinine)	1807	1883	1874
Henry Bowman Brady	1825	1891	1874
W. E. Forster (Right Hon., politician ; left Friends)	1818	1886	1875
John Gilbert Baker (keeper of herbarium at Kew)	—	—	1878
George Stewardson Brady, M.D.	—	—	1882
Sir Jonathan Hutchinson, M.D.	—	—	1882
Sir Edward Fry	—	—	1883
John Theodore Cash, M.D. ..	—	—	1887
Silvanus Phillips Thompson (electrician)	1851	1916	1891
Arthur Lister	1830	1908	1898
Joseph Jackson Lister	—	—	1900

TOTAL, 1851-1900 : 19.

Ralph Allen Sampson	—	—	1903
Francis Wall Oliver	—	—	1905
Joseph Barcroft	—	—	1910
A. S. Eddington	—	—	1914
L. Doncaster	—	—	1915

"Friends and the Learned Societies," article in *Journal of the Friends' Historical Society*, Vol. VII, No. 1, First month (Jan.), 1910, p. 30, and *Record of the Royal Society*, 3rd Edition, 1912. (Oxford University Press.)

That the proportion of Quakers elected F.R.S. was enormously greater than the proportion of the non-Quaker population so elected is proved by the following calculations.

The next table shows the total numbers of inhabitants of Great Britain who were elected F.R.S. from the foundation of the Society in 1663 to the year 1900. The numbers of Quakers and non-Quaker Fellows are shown separately and also the average Quaker and non-Quaker population during each period of fifty years. The nnmbers given for the Quaker population are, in two cases, guesses based on the statistics and facts previously given :—

Period.	Elections to Royal Society of		Average population of Great Britain during each period.	Probable average number of Quakers living in Great Britain during each period.
	Non-Quakers.	Quakers or persons of Quaker descent.		
1663-1700	449	4	5,500,000	40,000
1701-1750	728	8	9,500,000	?30,000
1751-1800	948	7	12,500,000	?20,000
1801-1850	1,296	17	22,108,000	17,000
1851-1900	817	19	33,642,000	17,000

From these figures we can calculate the rate at which Quakers and non-Quakers have been elected F.R.S. per million inhabitants. The results are as follows :—

Period.	Elections to the Royal Society per million inhabitants of	
	Non-Quakers.	Quakers.
1663-1700	81	100
1701-1750	76	?266
1751-1800	75	?350
1801-1850	58	1,000
1851-1900	24	1,117

If we take these figures at their face value, it seems that, between the years 1851 and 1900, a man had about forty-six times more chance of being elected F.R.S. if he was a Quaker or of Quaker descent than if he belonged to the general population.   Further, the rate of election of Quakers is so rapidly increasing, and the rate of election of non-Quakers is so rapidly decreasing, that, if we consider nothing more than the actual figures, we should have to anticipate that, at no distant date, the Royal Society will become a branch of the Society of Friends.   But any such conclusions are unjustified owing to the fact that the actual total numbers dealt with are so small compared with the total population. As Quakers are now " marrying out " more than before and as those who have left the community must be forgetting their Quaker ancestry to an ever increasing degree, it is probable that the number of full-blooded and recognised Quakers to be elected F.R.S. in the future will diminish.   But it is to be hoped that enquiries will be made and records kept of both partial or complete Quaker ancestry of Fellows elected in future years.

CHAPTER XVI

THE TEACHING OF MORALITY

Fanatical and reasonable morality—Use of religion in teaching morality founded on sentiment—Reasonable sins and fantastic sins—Use of moral prepossessions in balancing our brute natures—Evolution of ethics.

A thing that everybody knows and that nobody seems to realise is that morality based on sentiment is more compelling than morality based on reason. The man who is honest because honesty is the best policy is not so honest as the man who is honest for no reason at all. Thus there are two kinds of morality—fanatical morality and reasonable morality. Let us consider examples of each.

A Quaker travelling in a carriage with a lady was stopped by a highwayman who demanded his purse. This the Quaker gave up. The highwayman then asked his victim for his watch. The Quaker put his hand in his pocket and, failing to find his watch there, said he had left it at home. The highwayman then rode off. No sooner had he done so than the Quaker discovered his missing watch in another pocket. Instantly he stood up and leant out of the window shouting, " Hi ! Hi ! Come back ! I didn't leave it at home. Here it is." His companion pulled him back into the carriage by his coat tails and pacified him by pointing out that it was clearly providential that the man who had stolen the purse had been saved from the further crime of stealing the watch.

An Indian friend informs me that in the Laws of Manu, the oldest religious book in the world, it is laid down that one should never tell a lie except for two reasons, first to save one's life and secondly when paying compliments to a lady. This is an example of reasonable morality that appeals to everyone, which is more than can be said of fanatical morality. Mention has already been made of the remarkable success of the early Quakers in founding banks. Their contemporaries no doubt held the opinion that however little one wanted fanatical honesty for oneself, it was a highly desirable quality in one's banker.

To teach morality by pointing out the advantages of being moral is an appeal for reasonable morality and is a widespread practice. " Honesty is pleasing to God. I never knew a man lost in a straight road," said Sadi the Persian poet, thus suggesting an advantage in being honest. Bishop Butler in his well-known Analogy has a chapter on the moral government of God by rewards and punishments in which he points out the worldly advantages of being moral. In many religions " threats of hell and hopes of Paradise " are held out as stimulants to moral conduct.

But it is doubtful whether such appeals to reason are the best way of teaching morality to young children. A reasoned sanction for conduct tends to be weaker than a sentimental sanction because it is liable to be attacked and upset by reason. But if the child is taught a fanatical morality based on something in which conscious reasoning plays no part, if his morality is based on an un-reasoning adoration or love of something that is beyond his comprehension, then he will acquire, not reasons, but prepossessions in favour of doing good and against doing ill. " Profane reason " will make but little head-way against such prepossessions if they are sufficiently deep-seated. But such prepossessions have a yet more important function than to make us moral as will be explained in a later paragraph.

Fanatical morality has been taught and apparently can only be taught by means of religion. An example of the use of religion in giving a sentimental basis for morality is furnished by a book in my possession, written in the year 1851 by a Quaker lady (my maternal grand-mother) and entitled *Mama's Bible Stories*. In it may be found traces of the custom of human sacrifice, of taboo, of fetish and a primitive conception of the Deity, all admirably suited to a child's intelligence. Through-out the book one finds bad reasoning combined with admirable morals. Practically no motive is given for moral conduct except that it is pleasing to God. The moral sentiments in the book are never reasoned. They are mentioned incidentally. They are postulates, not reasoned propositions. Hence there is nothing in them likely to arouse reasoning on the part of the child and to cause them to become a reasoned part of his conscious-ness. They are therefore likely to reach the parts of the mind outside consciousness and thus to give rise to

influences that affect consciousness as moral prepossessions. This appears to be a reason why this mode of
teaching religious dogma is of value and why it is more
valuable the more it disregards the use of sensible
reasoning.

The child reads in the fairy story that the wicked
princess who tried to interfere with the marriage was
baked alive amidst general rejoicings. To the child
such a denouement is quite right and proper. To such
a child it is also right and proper that those whom God
does not love should be sent to hell. The child reads in
Mama's Bible Stories that God sent fiery serpents to bite
the people, that he sent a famine, that he told Abraham
to sacrifice his son Isaac without any regard for Isaac's
feelings, that Jonah, after his adventure with the whale,
preached to the people and made them sorry and " God,
therefore, did not punish them as he meant to do."
Such stories give the child a conception of the Deity as
something inscrutable, beyond reason and that must be
taken for granted. They are, therefore, an important
part of the process of producing moral prepossessions.
Hence it is that a religion purged of all crude and primitive
conceptions is necessarily far less suited for developing
the child's moral character than the book we are describing. The dawning mind of the child resembles that of
primitive man far more than it does that of a twentieth
century adult. Hence if we wish to produce in it moral
prepossessions, we shall do well to rely more on old
legends dating from neolithic times or earlier* than

---

* Flint knives are mentioned in the Bible (revised version) in
Joshua v. 2.

on any rationalised and modernised form of religious belief.

Religious belief may have value in education by its effect on the mind of the teacher besides on that of the child. The religious teacher will have a hatred and intolerance of wrong doing, which, because it is unreasoned, may powerfully aid the development of moral prepossessions in the child. Indians, for this reason, often send their children to be educated by Christian missionaries. They would regard conversion of their children to Christianity as a misfortune but they appreciate the value of the high moral ideals of the missionary on the developing mind. Whether they would not be better advised if they chose religious Indians to teach their children is a question well worth their consideration.

From the point of view of the educationalist the sole function of religion in education is to produce moral prepossessions. When once these have been produced the further teaching of religion, in many cases, is likely to do more harm than good. It is undesirable for the average child that his moral character should be hitched on to and depend on a creed that, later on, he may find to have little to do with the realities of life.

As the child grows up and changes into a more rational being, the teacher must rely on appeals to developing sentiments, such as self-respect and love of fair play. One of the uses of games and athletics is in developing the latter sentiment. The child's affection for and intercourse with other children gives opportunities for practicing moral conduct and thus of developing his moral character.

The above remarks apply to the average child. If however the child is naturally religious, the further teaching of religion is advisable. Such a child is likely to grow up into a man who will profess, and probably practice, a high standard of morality that, by tending to keep up the moral tone of the society in which he lives, is likely to be of use to others if not to himself.

It has been stated above that moral prepossessions have a still more important function than making us, or tending to make us, moral. We may discover what this is by looking round for a moment at contemporary life. We see that under the declining influence of religious belief, men's conduct nowadays partly depends on a standard of morality that they acquire from intercourse with their fellow men but also, in varying degrees, on what they consider expedient. The view that moral conduct is expedient naturally leads to the view that expedient conduct is moral and this again to the view that expedient conduct is what is expedient for one's self. The results of such hybrid morality are far from satisfactory. Theologians have distinguished between venial sins and mortal sins. This classification is out of date and we have now to distinguish between reasonable sins and fantastic sins.

" The youth who winked a roving eye, or breathed a non-connubial sigh," and who, in the play, "was thereupon condemned to die," was punished for a reasonable sin with which anyone in full possession of his faculties might sympathise. But what can we say about the Japanese firm who supplied large numbers of pencils to South African and Australian governments which contained only an inch of lead at each end, the rest of the pencil being solid wood, and who defended their fraud by the singularly feeble excuse that the pencils were up to sample ? This can only be described as a fantastic sin, for it was certain to be found out and certain to do harm to the guilty firm. The Germans in recent years, not only in commerce but also in the conduct of war and diplomacy, have shown a singular tendency to commit sins of this nature. An English man of business, who has had extensive dealings with Germans in Germany, says that " German firms which ten years ago would have scorned to do a mean thing, now unblushingly adopt all kinds of tricks in business. When caught, they bluster or smile weakly, offer some futile explanation, and promise to make amends. Usually their tricks are merely stupid and sure to be found out."* The character that all such tricks and sins have in common is that they are inspired by curiously short-sighted reasoning. In reasoning by a well-balanced mind, all the relevant data are taken into consideration one after the other and at length a correct judgment is reached. But we have seen that the process of considering the data is apt to be cut short if an unbalanced sentiment is present in the subconscious mind. The victims of the con-

---

* Quoted by Sir Percival Phillips in an article in the *Daily Mail* of 16th Sept., 1924. (See also note on page 144.)

fidence trick furnish a case in point. They suffer from short-sighted reasoning.

Psychologists tell us that our brute natures are vestiges of instincts that were of use to our animal ancestors.* In the well-balanced mind these instincts are held in check by acquired moral sentiments. The phenomena of fantastic sins further show us that our brute instincts, that belong to the subconscious part of the intellect, are only properly balanced by pre-possessions that belong to the same part of the mind.

It is not intended to imply that a morality based on reason uninfluenced by sentiment is not possible. On the contrary such a morality exists and a Twentieth Century Moral Code might be expected to contain such eminently practical maxims as the following :—

It pays to have good morals. But it also pays—and pays better—to have good manners. " Manners makyth Man."

Always show gratitude. It costs nothing and you needn't mean it.

A child learns to speak the truth. But when he grows up, let him put away childish things and learn to be tactful. The misfortunes of Joseph were caused by a lamentable want of tact.

In matters of conduct appearances are more import-

---

* According to McDougall, at the present time, " a school of reactionary psychologists " are trying to throw doubt on this view and to persuade us that the human mind is a *tabula rasa.* He says, " It suffices to appeal against this academic doctrine to the good sense and experience of mankind." (*Ethics and some modern world problems*, Methuen and Co., 1924.)

ant than realities. Hence modesty which conceals our feelings is a greater virtue than charity which displays them.

Self-respect consists in being polite to one's superiors and rude to one's inferiors. The man who is always polite is no gentleman. He is a dealer in second-hand motor cars.

Such rules, however practical they may be in every-day life, fail completely to act as moral prepossessions capable of balancing our brute natures. Those who lack such prepossessions are likely, when tempted, not to be level-headed but to be biassed by a preference for the more devious or more brutal of two alternatives. Thus we see that our moral prepossessions have a function yet more important than making us moral. They may fail to make us moral but yet be playing a valuable part in adding to our reasoning powers and in enabling us to treat the affairs of life with well-balanced minds.

Thus it is imperatively necessary in the education of the child that moral prepossessions should be developed, not only to give him a moral character but also to ensure that his sins—for sin he will—shall be reasonable rather than fantastic.

It has been said that from the point of view of the educationalist the sole function of religion is to produce moral prepossessions. This is not the only point of view from which the subject may be envisaged. McDougall in his *Introduction to Social Psychology* has expressed a doubt whether Western civilisation can survive the loss of its religion. He quotes with approval the views of Benjamin Kidd on this subject. The latter author says, in his book *Social Evolution*, that the motive force behind the long list of progressive measures carried out in England during the nineteenth century has " in scarcely any appreciable measure come from the educated classes ; it has come almost exclusively from the middle and lower classes, who have in turn acted, not under the stimulus of intellectual motives, but under the influence of their altruistic feelings." If we accept this statement it seems that we must also recognise that these altruistic feelings were the result of religious influence and habit combined with a very limited amount of education.

What is the source of the standard of right and wrong that we pick up from intercourse with our fellow men ? We were shocked when the German Chancellor referred to a treaty as a scrap of paper. This was an example of what we may call " lower expediency." But no one appears to have been shocked or surprised when a prominent English statesman was described, a few years ago, by a well-known writer, as being guided by the " higher expediency." Both kinds of expediency consist in regarding expedient conduct as moral or at least as praiseworthy. They differ merely in the degree in which such conduct differs from old-fashioned, narrow-minded, religious morality. A respectable man in whose education there has been no direct religious influence may, under favourable surroundings, lead a fully moral life in the sense that his conduct may be and, if he is not too much tempted, is likely to be up to the standard of morality of the society in which he lives. But the facts of contemporary history seem to show that this standard of morality, being due originally to religious influence, tends to deteriorate slowly in the absence of such influence. In other words, the loss of religious influence on society is a matter of serious import and several generations must elapse for the full effect of this loss to become apparent.

Another ground for suspecting that we need a leaven of sentiment in our mental outfit may be inferred from the probable course of development of moral character in our ancestors.

My experience of a number of monkeys kept by me for some time in captivity is one of the reasons why it is difficult for me to believe that our anthropoid ancestors possessed anything that could be regarded as a good moral character. W. J. Perry has brought forward reasons for believing that organised warfare on a large scale is a comparatively recent acquisition of mankind.* This may well be the case. But he goes on to suggest that our earliest ancestors existed in a state of primitive innocence, a thesis that he supports by very unconvincing arguments. " Is it true," he asks, " that an infant when in any way thwarted will evince anger, and start to make violent attempts to get its own way ? May it not be that it is reacting to the recollection of a former experience when, for example, it had been slapped by an angry mother, or had observed the process in the

* W. J. Perry, *War and Civilisation* (1917) and *The Growth of Civilisation* (1924).

case of an elder brother or sister ? " Such a question
is answered quite as seriously as it deserves by referring
to the story of the little girl who, when reproved for
fighting her brother, replied : " Satan told me to kick
him ; but spitting at him was my own idea."

It is highly probable that the pressure of population
on food supply was the original reason why our ancestors
left the shelter of the trees for the dangers of *terra firma*.
It is also probable that when they reached *terra firma*
they were still sufferers from a restricted food supply
and that they were in the habit of fighting each other
for it. The peaceable habits of certain existing savage
tribes are probably due to a loss of primitive pugnacity.
For instance, the Morioris, when driven from New
Zealand by war-like Polynesian invaders, took refuge
in the Chatham Islands where they lived undisturbed
for a thousand years. " In obedience to their teacher
Nunuku, benevolence to all was the predominating feature
of their ethics." In the year 1835, a party of Maoris
arrived and attacked them. " The loyalty of the
Morioris to the covenant of Nunuku was put to a severe
test. But, after some hesitation, they kept their faith
and offered no resistance. Hundreds of them were
killed ; the rest were enslaved, degraded, herded like
swine, and occasionally eaten like swine."* In the case
of another tribe of moral habits, it is recorded that if
one man has a grievance against another, he composes
a song about it, which he sings in public in the presence of

* *Reminiscences and Maori Stories* by G. Mair (Auckland;
Brett Publishing Company, 1925).

S

the aggressor. Such a custom is certainly not primitive. It is not a custom one would expect to find in a virile race. It seems probable that, in such cases, peaceable and moral habits are not due to moral character, that is to say to the power of controlling passions, but to a mental change in virtue of which passions have decreased in intensity.* In many primitive races customs are found which seem to be traces of primitive pugnacity. For instance, " According to Humboldt the natives of Guina detest all who are not of their family or their tribe ; and hunt the Indians of a neighbouring tribe, who live at war with their own, as we hunt game." In the opinion of the Fuegians, " a stranger and an enemy are almost synonymous terms," hence they dare not go where they have no friends, and where they are unknown, as they would most likely be destroyed. The Australian Black nurtures an intense hatred of every male, at least of his own race, who is a stranger to him, and would never neglect to assassinate such a person at the earliest moment that he could do so without risk to himself. In Melanesia, also, a stranger as such was generally throughout the islands an enemy to be killed. In Savage Island the slaying of a member of another tribe—that

---

* The singular insensitiveness to pain shown by native Australians appears to be an analogous racial abnormality. One has been known to cut off a toe in order to be able to wear a European shoe. Another having a wound in his foot remedied it by putting the offending member in a fire and burning it off. Whether such incidents are due to abnormal courage in bearing pain, or, as seems more likely, to abnormal obtuseness in feeling it, they indicate a condition of the nervous system which is certainly not primitive and is probably not useful.

is a potential enemy—"was a virtue rather than a crime." The early inhabitants of Palestine seem to have well understood the virtue of hating their enemies. In the Book of Judges (i. 4) we find an instance of the resulting brutality being punished by the Jews : " And the Lord delivered the Canaanites and the Perizzites into their hand : and they slew of them in Bezek ten thousand men. . . . But Adoni-Bezek fled ; and they pursued after him, and caught him, and cut off his thumbs and his great toes. And Adoni-Bezek said, Threescore and ten kings, having their thumbs and their great toes cut off, gathered their meat under my table : as I have done, so God hath requited me. And they brought him to Jerusalem, and there he died." At the time of this incident the Israelites used to exact tribute from the tribes they conquered. But at the commencement of their invasion of Palestine their habits were more primitive. They used to destroy men, women and children, and sometimes also the animals, in each of the cities they captured. The kings were taken alive if possible and afterwards were hung (Joshua iv. 24, 26).

If the foregoing description is true or partially true, then the view that our brute natures are vestiges of instincts that were of use to our animal ancestors appears to have an implication that does not, as yet, seem to have been recognised. We can most concisely consider what this is by imagining a discourse on morality by some Early Pliocene preacher to the following effect :—

" Being more fertile than your cousins the anthropoid apes, you suffer more than they do from a restricted food supply. Hence the feeling of hostility to strangers of their own species, to be seen in so many kinds of animals, has with you reached an extreme development. You have a feeling of hatred for any man you meet of another tribe. You wish to kill him and thereby prevent him from eating food that otherwise might be of use to you and your family. Your Miocene ancestors employed stones in settling their differences with strangers. But the need of fighting for your food has, in combination with other influences, sharpened your wits and you now use flint instruments in fashioning such lethal weapons as spears and clubs by which, under favourable circumstances, you may destroy a stranger with a single blow without the exertion and risk of a long drawn-out fight. This definitely establishes your superiority over the anthropoids and is the ultimate reason why, as the poet sings :

> ' Brutes do not meet in bloody fray,
> Or cut each other's throats for pay.'

" But as a result of living in a community, you have to curb this ' murder instinct,' which has become part of the instinct for self-preservation. In order to avoid the emotional tension that results from a repressed complex, your murder instinct must find another outlet. You have seen the singular ferocity with which a gang of monkeys—your distant relatives—attack other monkeys that trespass on its preserves. You must imitate them and, in place of robbing and murdering your fellows, you must join with your fellows in killing and robbing those members of

other tribes who rashly invade your territory. You
will thus develop a respect for property belonging to the
community, namely, the land on which it lives. This
is the fundamental virtue of patriotism. In fighting it
is necessary to obey your leader. Hence you have
developed another of the primitive virtues, namely,
respect for authority. The exigencies of social life have
led to yet another virtue expressed in the command,
'Thou shalt not steal from members of your own
community.' Each of these three primitive virtues
plays a part in balancing your brute natures. You may
safely use your reason in acquiring other branches of
knowledge, but if you 'eat the fruit of the tree of
knowledge of good and evil,' if you subject the sentimental basis of your ethics to the cold scrutiny of profane
reason, your mental equilibrium will be endangered,
so that in times of excitement your judgment is likely
to suffer. Of this danger, let enthusiastic reformers
beware ! "

At the present day, intellectual and large-minded
persons are dreaming of a wider patriotism that shall
embrace the whole of humanity. If the above description of primitive ethics is correct, this is an impossible
ideal, or at least one that can only be arrived at with
extreme slowness. A narrow irrational patriotism seems
to be necessary for our mental equilibrium. If it is
discarded, then, owing to the nature of what our narrow
patriotism balances or represses, it will be replaced not
by unpatriotism but by the bias of anti-patriotism. Thus
we find deeply engrained in human nature a serious

hindrance to our progress. This conclusion implies no justification for war or militarism. It is merely meant to assert that for one's mental equilibrium one needs to retain a preference for the interests of one's country that is based on sentiment and uninfluenced by reason.

THE END.

INDEX

Administrators as heads of departments, 43.

Administrator's method of deciding, 34.

Advertisements, 199.

Agassiz, 148.

Alexic theories, 178.

American war organisation, 130.

Annandale on university education, 124.

Antioch College, Ohio, 236.

Arabic language in education, 213.

Argon, discovery of, 186.

Armstrong, Sir William, 150.

Atlantic Cable, 133, 145.

Aurungzebe, Mogul Emperor, 228.

Authors, 162.

Avebury, Lord, 150.

Babbage, mathematician, story of, 6.

Baniya caste, 126, 210.

Bankers, 113.

Beaconsfield, Lord, 200.

Bessemer, Sir Henry, 150.

Bidder, G. P., his calculating ability, 55.

— — , his education, 117

— — , his power of factorising, 74.

Biffen on grading wheat, 27.

Bismarck, 199, 206.

Brunton, Sir Lauder, 167.

" Brute natures," 275.

Business instinct, 15, 138.

— — , lacking in experts, 109

Business men, careers of 16, 17.

Business men forgetting school knowledge, 16.

Business men's ignorance, 15, 18.

Buxton, 61, 72.

Calculating Ability, 53.

Calculators of deficient intelligence, 56.

Cardigan, Lady, 31.

Cat ranch scheme, 7.

Chess and draughts, 236, 237.

Chinese education, 205, 214.

Cinemas and music, 99.

Clark murder case, 31.

Classical languages in education, 205, 212, 216, 220.

Clemenceau on Lloyd George, 33.

Colburn, 54, 68, 75,87.

— , his life history, 90.

Commercial chemists, 137, 140.

Commercial travellers, 169, 201.

Committees, defects of, 41.

Common sense decisions by juries, 38.

— — — , nature of, 87.

Compliments, use of, 196.

Confidence tricks, 152.

Cooper, Sir Astley, 48, 172.

Cramming, 230.

Creative faculty of the mind as defect, 189.

Cricketer deciding subconsciously, 104.

Critical faculty, 192, 194.

Crookes, Sir William, 99, 190.

Cross-examination, 45, 51.

Darwin, Charles, 97, 190.

Dase, a calculator, 60.

Decisions, power of making rapid, 15, 20.

Diagnosis, rapid, 21.

Diamandi, a calculator, 60, 207.

Edison, 9, 13, 126, 130, 147.

Education and bankers, 113.

Education and business instinct, 110.

Education, changes needed in, 227.

Education, classical, 111, 205.

Education of commercial chemists, 140.

Education, scientific, 206, 218.

Engineers and education, 114, 116.

Englishmen as diplomats, 43.

Expert company directors, 18, 136.

Experts as administrators, 151.

Experts, consulting, 142.

Experts, mental processes of, 12.

Factorising, power of, 54, 74.

Ford's opinion of Edison, 148.

Forgetting, power of, 106.

Forgetting, practice in, 127, 114.

Forgetting unwelcome evidence 190.

Forgetting, use of, 110, 170, 192.

Forgetting school knowledge 16, 107.

Formal discipline, 232.

Formal reasoning, 103.

Fortune teller, 25, 31.

Fox and the grapes, Æsop's fable of, 177.

Fox, George, 238.

Freud, 2.

Galileo, 190.

General knowledge questions 237.

German banks, 143.

German commercial morality 144, 274.

German dye manufacturing companies, 140.

Globe-trotters, 164.

Guy, J. Q., on education, 115.

Hankin, G. T., on mental processes, 55.

Hawtrey, Sir Charles, 7.

Heine, 44.

Heblmholz, 104.

Higinbotham, on refusing credit, 26.

Hobbies, 231 (note).

Home work, possible bad effects of, 234.

Hoover, 131, 255.

Houdin, the conjuror, 60, 66.

Huxley, 136, 225.

Ignorance in business men, 15.

Imbecile calculator, 80.

Inaudi, a calculator, 72, 83.

Indian civilians, 108, 231.

Indian gentleman's views of English diplomats, 43.

Indians, memory of, 123, 124.

Ingenuity, 197.

Indigo, discovery of synthetic, 18.

Initiative, 116, 128.

Initiative and education, 235.

Instinct of statesmen, 32, 218.

Interest, ill effects of stimulating, 221, 222.

Intuition, 13, 74, 103, 118.

Inventors, 142, 161.

Isherwood, 117.

Japanese Education, 205, 214.

Jews and musical ability, 98.

Jones, Kennedy, 47.

Journalists, 46.

Judging character, 23, 30.

Jury system, 36, 177.

Jury system, legal opinions on, 50.

Jute mill, casual appointment to, 29.

Kaiser, The, 34, 35, 229.

Kelvin, Lord, 133, 135, 145, 183, 195, 197.

Keynes on Lloyd George, 32.

Kidd, Benjamin, 277.

Kitchener, Lord, 32, 48.

Koran, 213.

Krishna, L.K.A., 125.

Languages, effect of learning, 204, 206.

Lardner, on steam navigation, 174.

Leacock, Stephen, 114.

Levantines, 207.

Lister, Lord, 191.

Lloyd George, 32, 33, 217.

Macaulay, 42, 44, 180, 233, 239, 254.

Mahomedans, administrative ability of, 259.

Mahomedans, business ability of, 125, 126, 138, 213.

"Mama's Bible Stories," 270.

Mansfield, Lord, story of, 44.

Manu, Laws of, 269.
Mark Twain, 64.
Marwaris, 211.
Mathematics, teaching of, 237.
McDougall, 275, 276.
Meigs, Dr. C. S., on contagion, 182.
Memory, abnormal, 61, 64, 123, 127.
Memory, improvement of, 119, 85.
Memory of Indians, 124.
Memory of school knowledge, 107.
Mennonites, 255.
Mental arithmetic, 205, 209.
Mill, John Stuart, 223.
Mitchell, a calculator, 81, 90.
Montaigne's essays, 106, 132.
Moore, George, 123.
Moplahs, 126, 259.
Moral prepossessions, 270, 273, 276.
Morality, fanatical, 270.
Morality, reasonable, 269.
Morgan, A. E., 102, 118.
Morgan, Pierpont, 209.
"Mr. X," 23, 119.
"Mr. X"'s brother, 122.
Multiplication, 80.
Murder as a habit, 280.
Music and education, 101.

Napoleon, 237.
Neolithic legends in moral education, 271.

Neptune, discovery of, 186.
Newspaper propaganda, 195.
Noble, Sir Andrew, 150, 196.
Normal defects of the mind 35, 104.
Novel reading, 233.

Oliver, F. S., on German states men, 33.
Originality and memory, 132.
Overworking schoolboys, 129.

Parrot Memory, 208.
Parsees, 235.
Pitt, William, 108.
Plague, story of, 166.
Playfair, Lord, 175.
Pole, W., on Bidder, 74, 87.
Politicians, out-of-place, 35.
Precocity of musical genius, 92
Preconscious mind, 85, 86.
Pugnacity, primitive, 278.

Quadruplex Telegraphy, 9.
Quakers, 238.
—   , and railways, 252.
—   , and steam navigation 253.
—   , as bankers, 246, 269.
—   , chemists, 251.
—   , education of, 241.
—   , families, 245.
—   , honesty of, 268, 244.
—   , in iron industry, 253.
—   , numbers of, 244.
—   , philanthropy of, 256.
—   , scientists, 261.

Quakers, their shrewdness, 248.
——— , their success in business, 244.
Railways, opinions of, 173.
Raleigh, Lord, 15, 187.
Ramanujan, story of, 63.
Ramsay, Sir William, 187.
Rankin, W. M., 115.
Rây, Sir Prafulla, 124, 125.
Reasoning, formal or conscious, 103.
Reasoning on narrow range of data, 6, 236.
Recognising character, 23, 25.
Religion in education, 270, 272.
Religion, uses of, 277, 276.
Rhythm and multiplication, 81.
Rhythm and music, 96.
Roberts, Arthur, 196.
Roberts, Lord, 217.
Rumford, Count, 149.

Saer, on learning languages, 207.
Savages, mind of, 105.
" Schoolmaster's pets," 192.
Scripture, 63, 73, 204.
Scientific education, 206, 218.
Self-made men, 192.
Sherlock Holmes, 36, 48, 49.
Slavery, abolition of, 256.
Sleeping before deciding, 103.
Soaring flight, observations of, 28, 178.
Society of Friends, 238.
Spencer, Herbert, the philosopher, 4, 5, 116, 130.

" Spur of the moment," 2, 20, 104.
" Stage-coach common sense," 174.
Statesmen, their method of deciding, 34.
Stephenson, the founder of railways, 172, 176.
Stokes, Sir Gabriel, 1.
Subconscious judgment, 12, 21.
Subconscious mind, intellectual processes in, 9, 11.
Subconscious multiplying, 76, 83.
Subconscious mind, rapidity of its action, 29.

Tact, 191.
Tangye, Sir Richard, 249.
Telegraph operators, 126.
Telegraphist's devided attention, 68.
Thrionic phrases, 3.
Thugs, story of, 159.
Thurtell, a murderer, 51.
Travelling, use of, 170.
" Training one's eye," 28.
Typewriting, 104.

Vesalius, 184.
Vocational education, 11, 184.

Walker, Sir Gilbert, 178
Watt, James, inventor, 117.
Wells, H. G., 167.
Whitworth, Sir Joseph, 150.

Yarrow, Sir Alfred 117, 194.

Printed and bound by CPI Group (UK) Ltd, Croydon, CR0 4YY

01/11/2024

01782629-0009